Disease Selection
The Way Disease Changed the World

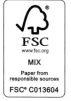

FSC
www.fsc.org
MIX
Paper from
responsible sources
FSC® C013604

Dedicated to Brian Southgate (1930–2011), my mentor and a great teacher, with whom I shared many of the interests contained in this book, which he would have loved to write if he were still with us. As a tribute I make him my posthumous co-author.

Disease Selection
The Way Disease Changed the World

Roger Webber

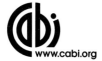
www.cabi.org

CABI is a trading name of CAB International

CABI
Nosworthy Way
Wallingford
Oxfordshire OX10 8DE
UK

Tel: +44 (0)1491 832111
Fax: +44 (0)1491 833508
E-mail: info@cabi.org
Website: www.cabi.org

CABI
745 Atlantic Avenue
8th Floor
Boston, MA 02111
USA

Tel: +1 617 682 9015
E-mail: cabi-nao@cabi.org

A catalogue record for this book is available from the British Library, London, UK.

Library of Congress Cataloging-in-Publication Data

Webber, Roger, author.
  Disease selection : the way disease changed the world / by Roger Webber.
      p. ; cm.
  Includes bibliographical references and index.
  ISBN 978-1-78064-682-4 (hbk : alk. paper) -- ISBN 978-1-78064-683-1
  (pbk. : alk. paper)
  I. C.A.B. International, issuing body. II. Title.
  [DNLM: 1. Communicable Diseases--history. 2. Host-Pathogen Interactions.
  WC 11.1]
  RA643
  362.1969--dc23

                                         2015020429

ISBN-13: 978 1 78064 682 4 (hbk)
          978 1 78064 683 1 (pbk)

Commissioning editor: Caroline Makepeace
Assistant editor: Alexandra Lainsbury
Production editor: Tracy Head

Typeset by SPi, Pondicherry, India.
Printed and bound in the UK by CPI Group (UK) Ltd, Croydon, CR0 4YY.

Contents

List of Illustrations

Preface and Acknowledgements

Diseases have been brought very much to the fore with the Ebola crisis, the recent epidemics of influenza and the more protracted concern of anti-biotic resistance. It is as though the problems of communicable diseases have come out of the cupboard to haunt us again. They were something of the past, within our ability to control and not something we need unduly concern ourselves with. This, however, has never been the case, as they have always been a problem in the developing world, where such diseases are an everyday fact of life. Just to survive malaria and diarrhoea has been a battle that most children have had to fight, while HIV (human immuno-deficiency virus) and tuberculosis are an ever-present threat to the adult. Much progress has been made and it is certainly a healthier world than when I first started out as a young doctor, but communicable diseases are still an ongoing concern.

When a current crisis is over we can put the problem of disease out of our minds. However, this is not what diseases are, something alien that comes to trouble us every now and then. They are part of our lives and, as will be seen further on, such an intimate part of us that they have more influence in our lives than we realize. They have taken a major role in making us humans and probably determine the way that we run our lives. To show this I have needed to start from the very beginning, from when life started, then as we emerged from our ancestral home in Africa, to carry our complement of diseases to the rest of the world. There followed the great epidemics that changed the history and demography of the world, which we survived because of our genetic variation and immune system.

So fundamental has been the part that disease has played in the world that it has brought about change, just as much as has natural selection. The purpose of this book is to show that disease has actually been another force, sometimes acting with natural selection but often in opposition; this is why the book is called *Disease Selection*. Appreciating the intimacy the disease process has with us allows for a greater understanding of its effects, enabling us to take preventive action and live healthier lives. If some of this happens then much of the objective of this book will have been achieved.

In order to cover the subject in breadth I have had to branch into fields of evolutionary biology, archaeology, history and others, in which at best I can only be an informed amateur. My resources have been the books by experts in the field and the boundless limits of the Internet. Even in just the medical literature, the number of references for each fact would be enormous, but taking in all the other subject areas, this is quite beyond the realities of compilation. I have attempted to list the main books and web sources used and many of the references will be found in them, with just a small number of the key scientific papers included in the resource material. This in no way reflects my lack of recognition for the considerable contribution by all the many who have advanced their fields of science. I hope they will forgive me for not quoting all their work in full. They have been a most valuable resource, for which I am very grateful.

I owe a particular debt to David Bradley for kindly going through sections of the manuscript and saving me from several errors. He has added considerably to my understanding of the processes of communicable diseases in the many years I have known him and I thank him for his continuing help. I apologize if I have still not got everything right, the fault for which lies entirely with me.

I would also like to thank Claire Allum for helpful discussions in archaeology and on the people of Africa. The origins of humans make up an ever-changing and controversial field, and her guidance in this has been most valuable, although many of the views remain my own. Everild Haynes has been the most excellent editor, not only in considerably improving the script but in adding her expertise in plant metabolism.

I am most grateful to CABI, the publishers of my textbook, who have allowed me to use several illustrations and tables from it, as well as offering every encouragement for this present work. This type of book is a new venture for them and I appreciate their confidence in me. For the other illustrations, I would like to thank the World Health Organization for permission to use Figs 4.4 and 7.3, Her Majesty's Stationery Office, London, for Fig. 1.2, Brainpicking.org for Fig. 7.2, and the Izikio Museum, Cape Town, the National Gallery of South Africa and the Blombos Museum of Archaeology for permission to take the photographs in Fig. 2.1. These and the other illustrations are provided freely for general use and as such are not covered by any copyright restrictions of this book.

Introduction

When Charles Darwin, with the often forgotten contribution of Alfred Russel Wallace, formulated the theory of evolution, it was the concept of natural selection that was to revolutionize an idea that had been discussed for some considerable time. The process of evolution had been understood, with the attempted explanation of Jean-Baptiste Lamarck (1744–1829) and even that of Erasmus Darwin, Charles Darwin's grandfather. But it was the paper written by Wallace on the island of Halmahera that, when it reached Darwin, galvanized him into action to elucidate in detail the theory that had been developing within him ever since his famous voyage on the *Beagle*, and resulted in the publication of *The Origin of Species by Means of Natural Selection* in 1859.

Darwin and Wallace had realized that multiple forms of creatures had been produced, but only those best adapted to the place and conditions in which they lived were successful and survived. Every place had specialist conditions, such as a particular food source, so that individuals would develop that were most suited to exploit this resource. These individuals would reproduce and the most successful of their offspring would fill this particular niche or expand into similar conditions under which they were more suited than the present occupants.

The development of modified individuals took place by a process of mutation in which changes to the genetic make-up would randomly occur. Many times these mutations were a disadvantage and the individual would not survive, but occasionally an improvement would arise that made the new individual more successful. Over considerable periods of time, small sequential improvements appeared to take place, although in reality they were a very extensive process of trial and error. In addition, during periods of stress, greater change has been found to happen due to the action of transposons (jumping genes), which greatly accelerate the process and often seem purposeful.

The natural environment would also change over long periods of time, new food sources would develop and circumstances improve or diminish, so that as these conditions changed then more suitable individuals would evolve to displace those that had been there originally. A new plant would originate that a new animal would find more edible or a prey animal would develop a defensive mechanism that protected it from its predator. Evolution was a continual movement; as one species changed it became more (or less) suitable for another species that fed on or otherwise benefited from it, and so the second species changed as well. Species were not fixed but changed over periods of time. Some were surprisingly successful, like members of the crocodile family that have remained in a similar planform for millions of years, while others, such as the flightless dodo, were no match for a rapidly changing environment and went extinct. In our rocks are to be found the fossilized remains of an incredible range of animals that were at one time successful, and sometimes extremely successful, like the trilobites, but in their turn were not the best suited for the prevailing conditions, and so became extinct.

Life then was a competition to be won by the fittest and most suited for the particular place and conditions. Success was judged not only by survival but the ability to pass on genes to the next generation. It might be the strongest male in a group of animals living in herds in which the dominant male had access to as many females as he could corral into his harem, such as with red deer, or the peacock with the largest and most beautiful tail that outshone his rivals. These were, however, risky strategies, as the dominant male in the herd would be challenged by rivals, who in time would overpower him, often with fatal consequences, and if the peacock had too large a tail it could not fly well enough to escape predators. A balance would therefore develop in which there was an amount of change that was the best fit for the purpose concerned, while at the same time not jeopardizing survival.

Darwin expanded upon the process in his second book on evolution published in 1871, *The Descent of Man and Selection in Relation to Sex*. The role of sex then became another process by which evolution took place, now generally known as Sexual Selection.

The term fitness is an all-encompassing term, to include the genetically most suited individual, with access to the best food source, as well as freedom from disease. A female bird will be able to tell from the sheen of the feathers whether a courting male has a burden of parasites, and a male herd animal obviously suffering from illness will not be strong enough to challenge the dominant male, so will be less fit. The contribution of disease can sometimes be out of all proportion to the other benefits that the individual may possess. The progeny may be the offspring of the best male and female in the flock or herd and brought up on the most advantageous source of food that its dominant parents can provide, but if it contracts an illness, this can put it at a disadvantage to its well, but genetically less suitable, rivals.

Changes in disease-causing organisms are produced in exactly the same way as the rest of nature is evolving, and provide a means for those organisms to dominate their environment. A parasitic organism is exploiting a niche by living on another organism, to its own advantage but to the other's disadvantage. This needs to be a compromise because if the parasitic organism is too successful and kills the animal it is invading before it has been able to reproduce, then not only will it be robbed of its food source but also of its ability to survive.

With virus infections, the virus is not a free-living organism, but depends upon the cells of its host to continue its existence, so the inevitable consequence is the demise of the host, or for the host to be changed so considerably that it is at a disadvantage compared with a healthy rival. To overcome viral infections, animals developed immune mechanisms that were able to eliminate the disease so that the animal was only temporarily incapacitated, giving it a greater chance to survive long enough to regain its previous vigour. Immune mechanisms have also developed against bacterial infections, and bacteria are in most cases self-contained organisms. These mechanisms would have been developed first as bacteria were the earliest forms of life on our planet (but see further in Chapter 1). Immune strategies have been developed against infections by most of the larger parasites as well, for instance the nematode worms, but these mechanisms are more compromising in allowing the parasitic organism to continue to live within the host organism without producing sufficient damage to kill it.

We have developed a very comprehensive immune system that originated with the reptiles some 300 million years ago. Both plants and lower animals have immune mechanisms, but it was not until the reptiles, and the subsequent development of mammals, that the type of immune mechanism we now have was selected by evolutionary processes.

Illness caused by disease is either part of the process of natural selection or, in some circumstances, directly opposes it. In HIV infection, it directly opposes natural selection.

In humans, to pass on his genes, the man needs to successfully mate with a woman, and natural selection encourages the male to mate with as many females as he is able or is permitted to by the female. The social constraints of marriage and moral standards modify this, but in history there are many examples, such as Genghis Khan or the Ottoman sultans, fathering huge numbers of children. Even within the constraints of marriage, in many countries large families were or still are the norm, to ensure sufficient surviving children to continue the family line. However, the more females a man mates with in HIV-infected areas, the greater the risk he has of developing HIV infection, so becoming debilitated and in course of time (modified by chemotherapy), dying from the disease. In other words, the more successful he is in endeavouring to pass on his genes the greater the chance he has in dying from disease, so disease is selecting against him.

Even if, as one of the preventive actions of combating HIV, monogamy is practised, the tendency of natural selection is directly opposed by disease selection. In many African countries, the major victims of HIV infection are women, most of whom have been in monogamous relationships. This is because their male partners have strayed from the relationship, often consorting with a high-risk sexual contact, so that they becomes infected and subsequently pass the infection back to their partner. If the woman becomes pregnant, then her infant is also likely to become infected, further opposing the process of natural selection to produce healthy children.

When HIV infection was first recognized and before control methods had been developed, some highly successful individuals that would have been key people in the development of their communities were the first victims. Highly successful individuals are often highly promiscuous as well – this is natural selection in operation – but disease killed them off. Zambia was one of the first countries to feel the full effects of the HIV epidemic, which killed a large number of successful business people and managers at all levels of society. This was to have a profound effect on the country, as disease has had throughout the ages.

Disease is often viewed as a temporary inconvenience, something that can be treated, and after it has passed, life continues again as normal. Even in epidemic form, it might kill off large numbers of people, but there are still others to take their place, and when the epidemic has passed, it is largely forgotten. But disease has had and continues to have a far more profound effect on all of us than has been realized; it has selected the course of the world just as much as the rest of nature has, as will be shown in the following chapters.

The Sexual Revolution

1

Origin of Life

The general consensus is that life originated in the oceans some 4 billion years before present from the heat and nutrients of hydrothermal vents. Although the heat originated from volcanic processes and was intense, it was cooled by the surrounding ocean and a gradient of temperature was created that provided the ideal conditions for life to start. This first life was very simple, just a cell wall containing cytoplasm, and could quite easily have happened, as shown by Wagner in his book *Arrival of the Fittest*; it was termed a prokaryote.

All cell walls are made from amphiphilic lipids, which are so called because one end likes water and the other likes oils and not water. This property enables lipid molecules to be directionally arranged, a phenomenon that is seen if a thin film of oil is spread on to water, in which it naturally forms into globules, thereby separating the oily components from the water outside. This is thought to be how simple cell walls originated, to be subsequently improved upon by random mutations of their organic contents.

These mechanisms enabled the development of two early life forms, the *Archaea* and the *Bacteria*, which set about colonizing the planet. Bacteria are found on all surfaces and in every part of the earth, even within rocks and thermal springs that are too hot for any other form of life. They have been found as far as 5.3 km down a borehole in Sweden, and in hydrothermal vents where they survive on sulfate and hydrogen, while one species known as *Deinococcus radiodurans* is able, as its name implies, to survive high doses of ionizing radiation, as well as being dried out and subjected to intense ultraviolet light.

Our bodies are covered with bacteria, they are in every orifice and happily live within our intestines (Fig. 1.1), providing us with almost 15% of extra calories from our food. Bacteria were so successful and in such abundance that for several millennia they and the *Archaea* were the only

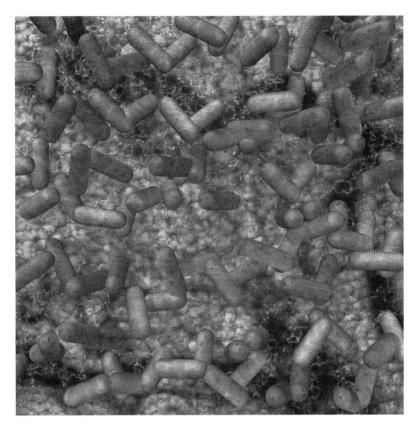

Fig. 1.1. A highly magnified picture of bacteria in the human intestines. (Reproduced with permission from Bluecrayola.)

forms of life on our planet, and there seemed no need for there to be any other. They were modified and became adapted to every place within our world (and possibly in other worlds). Yet, despite this abundance and variety, they reproduce in the simplest of ways – by dividing in half – in a process that is known as binary fission or asexual reproduction. (There are exceptions, with some bacteria using a modified form of sexual reproduction, but this only happens under certain conditions and in a minority of cases.)

Binary fission is a very easy process. First, a copy is made of the genetic material (chromosomal DNA), then the cytoplasm and cell wall divide, so that two identical organisms are produced. While this mechanism might seem applicable only to single-celled organisms, even multicellular life forms such as hydra can reproduce in the same way. Indeed, one might ask why, if reproduction can be achieved so simply, did animals develop two sexes and go through a complicated procedure to reproduce themselves? – a topic that is discussed below.

Even in higher animals though, there is still a surprising amount of symmetry within the body plan – two forelimbs, two hindlimbs, paired lungs and paired kidneys; and the heart has four chambers, one pair for receiving the blood and another for driving it round the body, which originally served each side of the body, but developed in mammals into a venous and arterial system for the whole body. It is almost as though the body could still be divided down the middle and each half then grow opposite parts.

Bacteria are far more efficient at reproduction than higher animals, not only in simplicity but also in rapidity, so that within a short space of time, favourable conditions allow the production of millions of them. However, it is this very success that is their weakest point because they are all identical. If there is something that can kill just one of them, then providing there is sufficient of that substance, it will kill all of them. When an advert claims that its product will kill 99.9% of germs it is probably correct.

None the less, random mutations do occur, so that in time a resistant strain could develop to the killer substance, and as every bacterium in that batch will be identical, all will have the same capacity of resistance. It is the rapidity with which bacteria reproduce that increases the chance of a beneficial mutation occurring. A single bacterium will produce a mutation at a rate of 10^4–10^9 cell divisions and if one of these should have an advantage, it will be selected and so become the predominant type. But if another lethal substance is used, all of the bacteria will once more be killed in an all or nothing process, there are not even a few that will survive to be the parents of a fitter strain. This is where sexually reproducing organisms have an advantage.

Animals with two sexes mix the genetic material from each parent so that there are numerous possible outcomes. Some individuals will be inherently weak and not survive to adulthood, while others will have a more suitable genetic make-up that enables them to be strong enough to survive and reproduce themselves. Some will have certain characteristics and abilities to withstand adverse environments while others will not. It was this necessity to survive the challenge from disease-producing organisms that led to the evolutionary selection of sexual reproduction. We are two sexes because we are more able to cope with disease that way. (This is a simplification of the original work done by Bill Hamilton, which is well described by Matt Ridley in *The Red Queen*.)

This challenge from disease came surprisingly early in life, with bacteria not only preying on each other but the mechanism of parasitism also appearing to have developed right from when life first started. Either one bacterium would invade another and live off its cell contents to the detriment of its host or it would be inadvertently engulfed, in the manner that an amoeba engulfs a foreign body, but not destroyed. From this position within the host cell, and providing that it survived, the bacterium could exploit the host cell to its advantage.

Viruses are incomplete life forms, needing the contents of a cellular organism to develop and reproduce, and they too have been found to have been present at the very early stages of life. Indeed, they might have been early attempts at creating life that were not able to complete the process. Every bacterium has a virus that preys on it, so the origin of disease, whether it be bacterial or viral, has been with us right from the very start of life.

It was this process of invasion of another bacterium, or that of being engulfed by one, that led to the most momentous development in life – the development of the eukaryotic cell. This is a more complex cell form than a prokaryotic cell, and contains a nucleus and other organelles; it is the basis of all multicellular organisms, both plant and animal.

The development of the eukaryotic cell was probably driven by attempts to develop new energy sources, particularly photosynthesis, that would free an organism from its dependence on chemical energy. But one of the consequences was the production of oxygen, which was like a poison to anaerobic bacteria. This not only changed the dominance of existing species but presented a continuing battle that is still with us today – how to prevent an excess of oxidants from building up in tissues. This topic will be covered in more detail in Chapters 15 and 16.

Evolutionary biologists have looked for some time for a suitable prokaryotic cell that when engulfed by another would form the nucleus of the nascent eukaryotic cell, but none has been identified that matches all the required criteria. However, Luis Villarreal, working with viruses, has come to the astounding conclusion that the primitive cell nucleus could have originated from a complex virus. The vaccinia virus, for example, seems to have all the same mechanisms that are required by a eukaryotic cell nucleus. The virus that formed the nucleus brought with it all the basic genes – thought to number about 324 – that are necessary to form the cell.

It requires a little time, and perhaps rereading of what has just been said, to realize that every cell in our bodies has a nucleus that was derived from a virus. We are the result of a very early disease process!

If this takes some getting used to, a fact of even more astonishment, and more generally agreed, is that some of the cellular organelles, particularly the mitochondria, could have been derived from parasitic bacteria. In the game of fleeing from threatening viruses, a bacterium might allow itself to be engulfed by another for protection, and if this set-up is sufficiently stable, then a symbiotic relationship will result. This is thought to have happened with a bacterium that subsequently became the powerhouse of all cells, the mitochondria.

One of the reasons we know that this happened is that mitochondria contain their own DNA, which means that the genetic make-up of mitochondria can be examined and compared with that of different bacteria to determine its close relatives. Drs Wang and Wu from the University of Virginia have just done this and come to the surprising finding that the inclusion bacteria (mitochondria) are more closely related to a parasitic ancestor that stole energy from its host, rather than giving it. They examined the pre-mitochondria (the earliest form and last common ancestor of currently existing mitochondria) and were able to predict that these possessed a plastid/parasite type ATP/ADP translocase that imported ATP from the host, so they were actually energy parasites. In addition the pre-mitochondria had a large number of flagellar genes, suggesting that the ancestor bacterium was likely to have been motile, and capable of oxidative phosphorylation under low oxygen conditions.

So not only is the nucleus of our cells derived from a virus but the mitochondria are from a parasitic bacterium. There can be no closer link between us and disease-producing organisms.

Coming back to the original discussion on sexual reproduction, this finding also helps to explain why there is such a disparity between the egg and sperm in human reproduction. Only the egg contains mitochondria, the sperm has just nuclear chromosomal (genetic) material and a flagellar mechanism that breaks off when the successful sperm enters the egg to fertilize it. The mitochondria were removed from the germinal cell that developed into a sperm, and there is no place for any other potentially pathogenic material to infect the egg during this conjugation. There is always the danger that the original bacteria, especially if there were two of them (one from the male and one from the female), could become pathogenic once more, so by removing the one from the male gamete this reversion is unlikely to take place. The cell is taking no risk that the early battle between the pre-eukaryotic cell and the invading bacteria should need to be fought again.

Complex Life

The invention of the eukaryotic cell took place about 2.2 to 1.8 billion years before present, and enabled the development of more complex life forms. There was then a period of over a billion years during which little happened, which led to one of the most dynamic periods in the development of life, the Cambrian explosion, some 542 million years ago. This is so called because of the profusion of new life forms that occurred over a brief period of time, although present-day thinking suggests that these developments might actually have occurred over a longer time scale. Early complex life forms were probably soft bodied and so left no imprint on the fossil record; it was not until the appearance of animals with external skeletons that we find fossil remains. The first of these to be found were the trilobites in the 1840s, but wider searches discovered stromatolites dating back to at least 1.4 billion years before present. These consist of algal mats related to green algae, and are significant because of their production of oxygen, which helped to provide the level of this gas in the atmosphere that we breathe today. Stromatolites can still be found in the shallow waters of Shark Bay in Western Australia.

This profusion of life led to the origins of many of the phyla which, apart from the bacteria and viruses, include all other forms of life that took on a parasitic type of existence and became the disease organisms that trouble us today. One of the earliest kingdoms to emerge included *Trichomonas* and *Giardia*, two important parasites of humans. Other relatively early parasites include *Plasmodium*, *Leishmania* and *Trypanosoma*, some of the most important of all disease-producing organisms.

These organisms not only exploited every niche of their environment but also found ways to live off the more complex animals that subsequently developed. This could either be to the advantage of the animal, as in the case of gut bacteria, which assist in breaking down food so that it can be digested, or to its disadvantage, as in the development of disease.

Natural History of Disease

When a new disease develops (from a random mutation or by transfer from another species) its effect on the animal it attacks will be severe. The animal has never met the organism before so it has never had an opportunity to develop defensive mechanisms and will either be killed or have a severe reaction. Such was the effect that the completely new disease severe acute respiratory syndrome (SARS) had on the first unfortunate human beings to meet this virus; out of the 8422 cases, there were 916 deaths and a number of survivors suffered chronic lung damage. If we had reproduced asexually like bacteria, then there would have been no survivors from those that had been infected, but because of the different genetic make-up of individuals, there were some that overcame the disease. One could hypothesize that if the disease had been allowed to run its course, then proportionally more people would have survived as they inherited defence mechanisms that made them more able to tolerate the organism. Fortunately, a major effort was made to eradicate SARS before it became a universal problem, but there are many other diseases that were not eradicated, with tuberculosis and leprosy being good examples of the natural progression of a disease.

Tuberculosis (TB) was one of the major killers of 19th century Europe, where it was known as consumption. This is in fact a very good description of the disease, as it gradually consumes the person who has it, the main clinical criteria being loss of weight and anaemia. As TB is predominantly a respiratory infection there is a persistent cough, often accompanied by the distressing symptom of coughing up blood, or haemoptysis. The infected person gradually wastes away, and generally has a long, lingering death.

Consumption spared nobody, wealth or ability being no barrier, and one of the most tragic examples was that of the famous literary family, the Brontës.

Patrick and Maria Branwell Brontë had six children, among them the famous novelists Charlotte and Emily. The first to die of consumption was the mother, Maria Branwell, and the two eldest children, Maria and Elizabeth, in 1821. The son, Patrick Branwell (fuelled by his addiction to opium and alcohol), expired in September and Emily in December 1848, a year after the publication of her famous novel *Wuthering Heights*. Emily's youngest sister, Anne, died in 1849 and finally Charlotte, in 1855 (Charlotte died during pregnancy, but it is likely that this was because she was consumptive).

Yet despite his wife and all his children dying from the consumption, as far as we know, the father, Patrick Brontë, never developed the disease. He had inherited resistance to TB (or had acquired immunity from early contact with the tubercle pathogen), which unfortunately was not passed on to any of his children. Gradually, the population of Europe inherited resistance to the disease, so that it ceased to be a public health problem before anti-tuberculosis therapy began to have any major effect, as seen in Fig. 1.2. Much of this decline was due to improved standards of living, but the innate resistance of most Europeans to TB is seen when they come into contact with high levels of the disease, such as when they work and live in developing countries.

There is a similar story with leprosy, which was the feared disease of the Middle Ages, when the afflicted person was incarcerated in some out

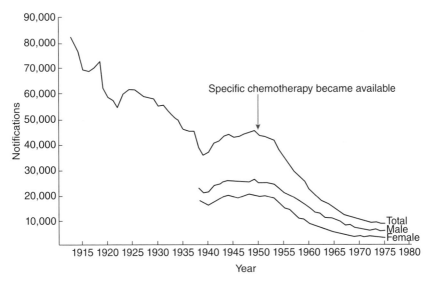

Fig. 1.2. The decline of tuberculosis (TB) in England and Wales in 1912–1975. From DHSS (1977) *Annual Report of the Chief Medical Officer, Department of Health and Social Security for 1976*, Her Majesty's Stationery office, London. Contains public sector information licensed under the Open Government Licence v3.0.

of the way place, forbidden to enter a tavern or church and required to ring a bell when walking, so as to warn people not to come near.

It is difficult to know where leprosy originally came from, but by 4000 BC it was already known in Egypt. Hippocrates described the disease in 460 BC and it is mentioned in the New Testament, with Christ healing cases. The disease also was known in China and India, where it was described in the *Charaka Samhita*, an ancient Ayurveda treatise written during the Gupta period (4–6th century AD). A pandemic in the 13th and 14th centuries, which originated in China, spread westward through India and Pakistan (where the Gupta Empire was centred) along the ancient trade routes (the Silk Road) to enter Europe. Even kings were stricken down by the disease.

Robert I, or Robert the Bruce (1274–1329), King of Scotland, suffered from leprosy, as was confirmed by finding bone changes to his skeleton when his tomb in Dunfermline Abbey was opened. This is further supported by the story that when he visited St Fillan's Church in the grounds of Aberdour Castle, he looked through the leper's window, as even a king with leprosy was not allowed inside. St Fillan was also called 'the leper', as he either had leprosy or a deformity of his right arm which was considered to have magical powers. Robert the Bruce had come to the church to take the holy relic (the arm bone of St Fillan encased in a silver casket) into battle with him and perhaps hoped that it would rid him of leprosy as well. It did bring him success against England in the Battle of Bannockburn in 1314, but did not cure his leprosy.

Henry IV of England, or Henry Bolingbroke, may also have had leprosy, but this is more in doubt. The strongest candidate for the title of 'leper-king' goes to Baldwin IV (1161–1185), King of Jerusalem. In his youth he was found not to suffer any pain in his arms, and then signs of lepromatous leprosy took hold and led to his early death at the age of 24. Despite his affliction, which was added to by suffering from corneal ulceration leading to blindness, he was able to hold Jerusalem for the Christian Crusaders, although on his death it fell to the forces of Islam.

Leprosy is a spectrum of disease complexes dependent on the response of the individual to the invasion by *Mycobacterium leprae*, with lepromatous leprosy at one end of the spectrum and tuberculoid leprosy at the other. Lepromatous leprosy reflects the complete breakdown of the person's immune response, with bacilli present in the skin, leading to progressive damage to the nerves and the tissues they serve, while tuberculoid leprosy exhibits such a strong immune response that no organisms are found and damage is produced by the severity of the host's response. In between these two types is borderline leprosy, in which the disease can progress to either the tuberculoid or lepromatous side of the spectrum.

For hundreds of years it was assumed that it was skin contact with an affected person that caused the transmission of leprosy, hence the policy of the church to ban lepers from buildings and from narrow passages where they might bump into someone, and to warn people to keep out of their way. Only recently has it been discovered that leprosy is not transmitted by direct contact. During active disease, bacilli congregate in the nose, and it is droplets from nasal discharges, which are able to survive for 2–7 days outside the body, that are the important factor, with probably repeated infection or a large infective dose of organisms required before another person becomes infected.

By the early 20th century leprosy had all but died out in Europe due to the development of resistance in the population. However, this was not the case in the rest of the world, as will be discussed later.

Two Sexes

So from the above, we can conclude that the development of sexual reproduction had an advantage in producing individuals that were resistant to disease, and that in time resistance spread through the population. In this way, it was the constant attack by disease organisms acting as a driver that selected individuals – individuals that had been produced by a male and a female.

Out of Africa

2

Human Origins

In most maps of the world, Africa appears in the middle. This is purely a cartographic convention, as Africa is immediately below Europe, where map-making originated and the prime meridian of longitude was aligned with Greenwich, UK, in the international conference of 1884. However, this result is more than chance, as in many ways Africa is the centre of the world, because it is divided more or less horizontally by the equator, and in the original supercontinent of Gondwana the nascent Africa was at the centre of the land mass, with all of the other continents separated from it. The remnants of this division can be seen in the west by the mid-Atlantic ridge, with the Americas still moving westwards, and in the east with the separation of Madagascar, India and Antarctica (which subsequently moved south). Arabia is currently moving away from the Horn of Africa to ever distance itself from once being part of the African continent.

Many of the ancient plants and animals had their origins in Africa, the best documented of these being our own species *Homo sapiens*. The search for the missing link between apes and early humans still continues, with contenders found in Ethiopia, Chad, Kenya, Tanzania and South Africa, but what is certain is that it was in Africa that the human species originated.

The origin of humans probably occurred some 5 million years ago when global climatic change locked up so much of the planet's water that even the Mediterranean was drained, robbing Africa of its source of moisture and changing the equatorial forest into fragmented woodland and savannah. This meant that forest dwellers would have had to spend more time on the ground, thus forcing evolutionary change on to a now predominantly ground-inhabiting ape. Two groups evolved, one that kept to the forest and evolved into the chimpanzee lineage, while the other learnt to exploit the open areas between the woodlands, and in time adapted to walking on two feet.

Another change in the climate occurred from 3 to 2 million years ago in which the forest shrank further, favouring those early apes that had exploited the open ground. Two adaptations developed, one that continued with a vegetarian diet and the other that ventured into eating scraps of meat and bone marrow remaining from kills made by large predators. Although this latter species, called *Homo habilis,* had tool-making capability, it still retained many apelike features, except for its expanded cranium. Chimpanzee brains have a volume of 400 ml whereas estimates derived from the fossil remains of *H. habilis* range from 600 to 800 ml. Why was there this difference? It could not have been due to tool making or warfare, as chimpanzees are able to engage in both of these without having a large brain. What is certain is that having a bigger brain was the defining characteristic that led to the human race.

Many theories have been proposed as to why the brain, in what was to become the human line, should develop to such an extent. There were clearly disadvantages in having such a large skull, as it placed undue strain on the female pelvis during delivery, and required that the infant be delivered at a much earlier stage than in chimpanzees or other animals, which meant that it then needed constant attention and care for a longer period. With such disadvantages, there must have been considerable factors favouring a large brain; could it be that it was essentially due to sex? While the competition between males (and between females) is a continual striving to outdo others, the relationship between a man and a woman that is required in courtship is an even more powerful driver. The greater the cerebral ability, the more intricate the strategy used to attract the opposite sex and, equally, the greater the requirement of the opposite sex to win favour. Factors such as these could have pushed evolution to favour the bigger brain, and if the main driver was indeed sex, then as has been argued, separate sexes were driven by disease. Could it then be that the challenge to humans from disease, which led to separate sexes, also led to us having larger brains?

The development of the brains of animals is due to the action of specific genes, but the process appears to have been speeded up in humans to allow the brain to develop at a greater rate. The mechanism by which this takes place seems to be via transposons (jumping genes), which are particularly active in brain development. These genes are able to jump from one place to a more targeted part of the brain cell to insert genetic material where it will have the greatest effect. This is a process that particularly shapes the variety and personality of the individual. Recent work by Liana Fasching and a team at Lund University in Sweden has shown that retrotransposons or human endogenous retroviruses (the HERVs mentioned in Chapter 3) are responsible for the regulation of which genes are expressed in the brain, and why brain cells are so dynamic and multifaceted. The infection by these retroviruses that occurred is probably very ancient, but in the newly evolved human, they took on a remarkable facility to promote brain development.

Some 1.7 million years, ago a new human species (variant), *Homo erectus*, evolved, presumably descended from *H. habilis*, and characterized by more human-like features, with the male and female being of more similar size. There is also a suggestion in *H. erectus* of the origins of the male/female shared society that is characteristic of humans, rather than the separate male and female hierarchies found in chimpanzee societies.

The wandering *H. erectus* had adapted to living in dry places, which allowed it to migrate from Africa. One descendent of *Homo erectus* reached Asia, where stone tools found in northern China dated its presence there to at least 1.66 million years ago. Another migrated to Europe where, according to the view of Chris Stringer, it evolved into *Homo heidelbergensis* some 500,000 to 600,000 years ago. *H. heidelbergensis* then went through an evolutionary split around 300,000 to 400,000 years ago. In western Eurasia, one line developed into *Homo neanderthalensis* under the pressure of returning glacial conditions. The other line, in Africa, developed into modern *H. sapiens* about 150,000 years ago, probably in a small area of East Africa.

Remains of *H. sapiens* have been found in many parts of Africa and these early humans developed cultural advances that we can identify with modern humans. In Blombos Cave in Western Cape Province, South Africa, for instance, a 100,000 year old chemistry assemblage was found for mixing ochre that was used to adorn the body and possibly to make cave paintings (Fig. 2.1a,b). Drilled shells showed traces of red ochre powder from body paint, and polishing around the holes caused by rubbing against a leather or fibre cord showed that they had been strung together as a necklace (Fig. 2.1c.). The ochre had come from a different place, suggesting that trade had taken place and, intriguingly, had scratched designs on it (see Fig. 2.1b), the earliest representations of art.

Skeletal remains of these early South Africans are consistent with the present-day Khoisan people, who used red ochre for hunting and exorcism ceremonies, as shown in the many rock art sites found in southern Africa. Disease was regarded as evil spirits that needed to be cast out and one wonders whether this appreciation was also present in the people that inhabited Blombos Cave.

Further along the coast from Blombos Cave, at Pinnacle Point, are caves that contained evidence of fishing and of beachcombing for seafood some 100,000 years ago (Fig. 2.2). An even earlier site was found at Klasies River Mouth in the Eastern Cape Province of South Africa, which was dated to 140,000 years ago, and another in Eritrea at Abdur (on the Red Sea coast not far from the later Axumite port of Adulis), which was dated to 125,000 years ago. At Abdur were found Middle Stone Age tools and shellfish remains mixed with larger animal bones in shell middens. These findings have led to a realization that the exploitation of aquatic resources might have been a strategy that was used by people when they

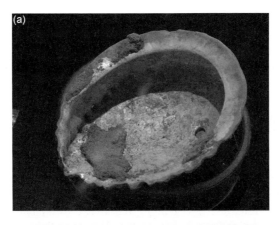

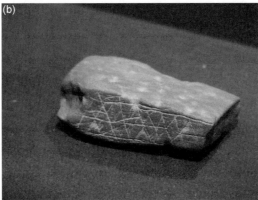

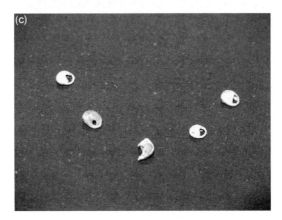

Fig. 2.1. (a) 100,000 year old shell used for mixing ochre, (b) an engraved block of ochre and (c) pierced shells from a necklace, all found in Blombos Cave, South Africa, and indicating modernity in humans. (Pictures taken with the permission of Izikio Museum, Cape Town, the National Gallery of South Africa and the Blombos Museum of Archaeology.)

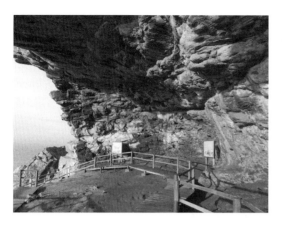

Fig. 2.2 An excavated cave at Pinnacle Point, South Africa, where the use of beachcombing and fishing from 100,000 years ago show how this might have been the way humans migrated round the world.

were migrating around the world, especially in places where deserts or the sea made crossings dangerous. Unfortunately, with the various changes that have taken place in sea level as a result of past climate change, most coastal sights have been destroyed.

Considerable discussion has taken place as to where it was that *H. sapiens* left Africa, either by a northern route across the Sinai, or by a southern route to (modern) Yemen across what is called the 'Gate of Grief' – the strait that separates the lower end of the Red Sea from the Gulf of Aden, or even by both routes. The southern route implies the use of watercraft, as even at the time of maximum Ice Age freezing, sea was always present in the strait. This would have been quite a momentous step for an animal that had only recently developed elemental technologies – and a step for which we have no evidence. Although it would have taken much longer, *H. sapiens* could just as easily have left Africa by following the coast northwards right round the Red Sea until these early humans reached the Arabian side, eating seafood as they went. At different times, some could then have taken off on a more northerly route while others continued round the coast on their way eastwards.

Expanding all the time, this initial group of travellers probably eventually reached India, where it divided into two. One group followed the coast of South-east Asia to arrive in Australia some 60,000 years ago. The other group headed north-west, reaching Europe around 45,000 years ago, where they gradually displaced (as well as intermixed with) the Neanderthals, to expand into the cold northern latitudes of Eurasia. The next ice age episode of 20,000 years ago drove these people south, and then their descendants, returning with the retreating ice and probably following herds of reindeer, found the land bridge that allowed them to travel into the Americas from Siberia.

While this pattern of migration generally seems to be the case, genetic evidence reported by Cann, Stoneking and Wilson in 1987, although supporting the fossil record, suggests that the migration from Africa was a precarious event. This conclusion is based on the examination of mito-chondrial DNA, which is inherited only by females, and showed that all of us originated from a single female who lived some 10,000 generations (150,000 years) ago, generally dubbed 'The African Eve'. Of course, she must have had a mate and there were others in her group, probably some 5000, although the number could have been as low as 150, but these fe-males lost their genetic influence by having only sons or non-fecund daughters.

On reaching Eurasia, these early *H. sapiens* met members of the pre-vious human variant to leave Africa, *H. neanderthalensis*, and bred with them some 50,000–60,000 years ago, as all Europeans and Asians contain 2% of Neanderthal DNA. The two continued to live alongside each other, but the distinctive Neanderthal died out about 30,000 years ago. We there-fore possess features of these early human species and their demise might be viewed as more of an absorption rather than a displacement. What is even more intriguing is the discovery of other ancient DNA remnants that could indicate that some inbreeding took place with *H. heidelbergensis* as well.

The original Neanderthal DNA sample was extracted from a finger bone of an adult female living in the Denisova Cave in the Altai Mountains of western Siberia. Also living in the cave was another species of human, who have been called the Denisovans, with whom the Neanderthals also bred. Some 3–6% of the Denisovan genome came from breeding with an unknown group of archaic humans, with the possibility that this could have been *H. heidelbergensis* or even *H. erectus*. (As an aside, up until the discovery that *H. sapiens* had bred with *H. neanderthalensis* and possibly even with *H. heidelbergensis* or *H. erectus*, these were all regarded as sep-arate species. However a species is defined as a group of animals that are able to breed with each other but not with organisms of other groups, so they should in fact all be regarded as variants belonging to the same species. We should probably call our own species *Homo heidelbergensis sa-piens* or *Homo erectus sapiens* (*H. h. sapiens* or *H. e. sapiens* for short) and the Neanderthals *Homo heidelbergensis neanderthalensis* or *Homo erectus nean-derthalensis* (*H. h. neanderthalensis* or *H. e. neanderthalensis* for short), but I will leave the experts in scientific nomenclature to decide on this.

While they were determining the mitochondrial DNA of different ra-cial groups around the world, the geneticists found a much greater vari-ation within indigenous groups in Africa than they did in other parts of the world. In other words, there was more genetic variation between two individuals from Nigeria than there was between a Norwegian and a person from New Guinea. From this, it can be concluded that life in Africa was not only difficult, but a matter of survival, and that when once free of the continent, life was not only easier but a rapid expansion took place. It was as though the cork had been taken out of the bottle and its contents could then explode into a vacant space. So why was it so much easier? Was it due to a greater preponderance of foodstuffs or to a more favourable climate, or was it escaping from the greatest slayer of the human race, disease?

When *H. sapiens* migrated from Africa, Europe and much of Asia was covered in ice, making conditions in the northern part of the world quite inhospitable. *H. neanderthalensis* occupied much of this area, so there would have been competition and resentment of the new invader, although as mentioned above, inbreeding did take place. While *H. sapiens* did finally dominate, initially *H. neanderthalensis* would have been in the majority and it would seem more likely that the powerful Neanderthal males might well have attacked *H. sapiens* and taken their females to mate with them, rather than the other way round, as is generally presumed. One advantage that *H. sapiens* might have brought out of Africa was immunity to several diseases, with the not unreasonable assumption that they also brought the diseases as well – much in the same way that missionaries took diseases to Pacific islands and Spanish invaders did to South America, as mentioned below. Smallpox and typhus do not leave marks on the skeleton so we cannot tell whether an infectious disease decimated *H. neanderthalensis* and contributed to their final extinction. Perhaps it was disease not just the superior intellect of *H. sapiens* that led to the demise of our closest human relative.

This theory is supported by calculations of the origin of body lice (*Pediculus humanus corporis*), made from analyses of their mitochondrial DNA, to around 80,000 to 170,000 years ago. Originally an ectoparasite of chimpanzees from some 6 million years ago, the louse transferred to humans as our species diverged. Not only does this indicate the use of clothes and bedding (to which body lice attach their eggs) by modern humans in Africa, but also that these humans carried the vector of typhus – the body louse – with them. Typhus comes in epidemic form, as discussed in Chapter 4, and when it spread to *H. neanderthalensis*, who would have had no immunity, could have had a devastating effect.

Typhus can persist in people, with the organism remaining dormant in their bodies long after they had the illness, a condition known as Brill–Zinsser disease. Cases have been found 20 and 40 years after the person was in a typhus area, but when particular conditions cause a breakdown in their resistance, then overt disease reappears. By this means, typhus could have been carried out of Africa to be subsequently transmitted to Neanderthals.

Agriculture was not discovered until some 10,000 years ago, so early man was still a hunter–gatherer, which limited family size to the area that could be foraged, as happens with the hunter–gatherer groups still remaining today. From studies of these groups, it has been calculated that on average each person requires one square mile of foraging area, or in other words a family group of five requires five square miles. Very soon there is a limit to the size of area that can be foraged by an increasing population, and new groups have to split off or population size has to be controlled. So although population size was not great, *H. sapiens* would have found large areas already occupied by Neanderthals.

Hence, there was no bonanza of food, the climate was not particularly favourable and there were other human ancestors competing for survival. Could the rapid expansion of early humans then be an escape from disease?

The First Diseases

Africa is the disease capital of the world. Many of the diseases that are found there are in no other continent, such as *Trypanosoma brucei* and its two human forms, *T. b. rhodesiense* and *T. b. gambiense*, which cause African sleeping sickness. Then there are the parasitic worms that have now spread to other parts of the world (see Chapter 7, The Slave Trade in Parasites) or have been given their names, such as Guinea worm, from the part of Africa from where they were first found. Even in recent times, the deadly diseases of Ebola and Lassa haemorrhagic fevers have come out of Africa. Human immunodeficiency virus 1 (HIV-1) originated from chimpanzees and HIV-2 from Sooty Mangabey monkeys, both in Africa, and malaria almost certainly originated in Africa.

As there is a bird malaria and one that infects reptiles it can be assumed that the ancestor of the malaria parasite is at least 130 million years old, as this was when these families diverged from the dinosaurs. The malaria parasite now known as *Plasmodium* probably originated 60 million years ago when it inhabited the guts of reptiles. The parasite was then transferred to mammalian predators, where forms evolved that entered the bloodstream. At some time, it adapted to the *Anopheles* mosquito, by which it was more easily transmitted. The antiquity of the parasite can be shown by the development of distinct species in different kinds of mammals that cannot infect animals of a different species, e.g. *P. berghei*, the rodent malaria parasite, does not survive if transmitted to humans. (This scenario would seem to be the logical explanation from the evidence we have, but because the sexual stage of the *Plasmodium* life cycle takes place in the mosquito, it might be that malaria is actually a disease of *Anopheles* mosquitoes that infects mammals as an intermediate stage.)

P. falciparum is the most severe form of malaria and is thought to have originated in West Africa as it has a close genetic similarity to *P. reichenowi*, the chimpanzee malaria parasite. The two species diverged some 10 to 4 million years ago, as estimated using the genetic clock technique (counting back the number of generations that are likely to have taken place for each mutation), dates that approximate with those from the archaeological evidence.

For some time it was thought that one of the human species of *Plasmodium, P. vivax,* originated in Asia, as its closest genetic relative was found in Asian macaques, while the other relatives were African. Recent work, however, has found a more closely associated *P. vivax* genetic sequence in faecal samples from chimpanzees and gorillas, suggesting that this parasite also evolved from a single ancestor that subsequently spread out of Africa.

It is difficult to trace back the origins of other diseases, but malaria and those infections restricted to Africa had their origin there, and it is quite likely that many others did as well. Diseases that evolved with early humans must have originated in Africa, putting pressure on our species as one of the factors that led to early humans taking the momentous step to leave the continent. As the original site of many of the diseases that afflict humans, Africa still retains its capacity to be the most deadly part of the world.

Sleeping sickness was probably particularly important, because it would have had a marked effect on the early hunter–gatherers. The bushbuck is commonly infected with *T. b. rhodesiense* so the ranging tsetse fly would feed on both bushbucks and humans, thereby transmitting infection. For an adult hunter from such a small group to be infected was a serious problem and if several were infected at the same time, which could have been quite a common occurrence, it would have been a fatal or certainly a debilitating blow to the whole of the hunter–gatherer group. Although *T. b. gambiense* does not have an animal reservoir, it is thought to have originally been a parasite of forest-dwelling apes and possibly pigs, so might have been as serious to hunter–gatherer groups as *T. b. rhodesiense.* Of course, we cannot be sure at what stage trypanosomiasis became an infection of humans, but knowing how readily diseases of animals transfer to humans (Chapter 12), it seems highly likely that this was early on in the development of our species.

Africa would have been covered in a mixture of forest and savannah, an ideal habitat for the various species of tsetse flies. Even if it had not yet become the vector of sleeping sickness, there would only have been a few places where humans could have escaped the ferocity of this fly's bite, with the extremes of the continent – the south and the north – being the main ones. There is a limit to how far south one can go, but going north and following a coastal route would have avoided this 'Curse of Africa'. There seems good reason to presume that disease, in particular sleeping sickness (or its vector the tsetse fly), encouraged early humans to leave Africa and find their way into the rest of the world.

The hunter–gatherer, or the preferred term of forager, acquired a considerable knowledge of local plants that they could eat and so help to relieve some of the symptoms of diseases. This knowledge was passed on from one generation to another, and the breadth of understanding of local fauna and flora that was acquired continues to amaze experts who study remaining groups of these people today. However, learning about medicinal plants and substances goes back even further, to at least our ape ancestors. Red colobus monkeys in Zanzibar are very fond of a particular leaf which forms the main part of their diet, but it also contains poisonous substances, so they have learnt to raid the local charcoal ovens and eat charcoal at the same time so that the constituent poison is deactivated. Chimpanzees have been observed to seek out a certain plant that probably cures them of worm infections. It seems that the ability to treat ourselves has been with us for a long time, and similarly originated in Africa.

Genetic Diversity

The effect of leaving Africa is shown by the reduced amount of genetic diversity in the people that came to inhabit the rest of the world. So was there an advantage in having a greater diversity of genetic material?

If two related people have children, then the pool of genetic material from which they are able to pass genes on to their children is limited. This is shown in some families in which notable genetic traits, such as the Hapsburg lip of the Austria–Hungary royal family, was passed on from generation to generation. Sometimes there is a lethal condition, such as haemophilia, and because of the dangers of closely related people producing children, most religions refuse to allow marriage between immediate family members.

So some genetic diversity is an advantage, and the greater the diversity of the gene pool the more variety there will be in the traits of individuals in that population. With this greater variety, there are more traits for natural selection to act upon to select the fittest individual to survive. This will be advantageous in combating new diseases or new variants of disease (such as the influenza virus) that have not been met with before. In an existing disease, the immune mechanism will already have made antibodies to combat the infection or, if over a long period, genetic modification will have taken place to confer resistance.

In Africa, the pressure of disease has selected for the most (genetically) diverse individuals. This is seen in the original tribal groups, with the greatest genetic diversity so far measured in the San or Khoisan of the Kalahari. The Bantu people, who originated in West Africa near to what is now the Nigeria/Cameroon border, displaced the original inhabitants as they progressed south, meaning that the people of southern Africa were there long before the present-day majority population of South Africa. Such was the genetic diversity of the original tribal groups that samples taken from four San in different parts of the Kalahari had greater differences from each other than an average European does from an Asian, yet in all outward appearances of physical characteristics and colour they appeared to be identical.

Because genetic diversity has an advantage, there is no value in restricting breeding to selected groups based on race or colour. Indeed, there is considerable advantage in genetically diverse groups producing offspring. Also, genetic diversity not only confers advantage in protection from disease but has permitted greater opportunities for other advantages as well.

Namibia is a particularly interesting country in this respect, not just because many of the Kalahari and hence the San people are within its borders, but because of an unexpected social experiment that took place there. Originally called 'South-West Africa', this part of southern Africa was in German possession during the colonial period, and became a refuge for a mixed race of Khoikhoi (Nama)/Afrikaner people, known as the Basters, who were discriminated against in South Africa. In the early 1870s these people were led by Hermanus van Wyk to Rehoboth, home of the Bondelswart Namas, in what is now central Namibia. They have a similar physique to the San, but speak Afrikaans and must be one of the most genetically diverse peoples anywhere in the world. When I visited Rehoboth in 1985, I was amazed by the beauty of the people, they were some of the most attractive I had ever seen.

Now we are quite used to people of mixed race and they have more than proved the advantage of diverse genetic couplings – as actors, sportsmen, lawyers, doctors and of course politicians – up to the highest office of President of the United States. It is tragic that the misguided ideas of fascism and racial cleansing are still with us, and indeed even the less extreme of nationalism, or the favouring of certain racial groups. These perpetuate a limited gene pool which in time may have insufficient alternative genes to cope with a challenge to that society (such as a new disease). Conversely, multiracialism has every advantage, both for increasing the genetic fitness of the population to disease and in the variety of individuals that are available to serve the society in which they live.

Disease Selection and Race

The selection for paler skin colour was probably due to the need for vitamin D, which prevents the disease conditions of rickets and osteomalacia. As melanin protects the skin from the more damaging effects of sunlight, which includes the destruction of folic acid in the body by ultraviolet light, a dark skin colour was an advantage in the tropical regions of Africa. But once early humans had migrated to northern climes, the presence of melanin would have prevented the conversion of cholesterol to vitamin D in the more subdued light found there. Here, it is pertinent to note that one gene, *SLC24A5*, is responsible for 30% of skin colour difference.

Natural selection then favoured racial separation, with lighter skinned people in the northern cooler climates and darker skinned people in the hotter regions near the equator. In contrast, disease selection favours those of greater genetic diversity and the mixing of different racial groups.

Host/Parasite Interaction 3

Effect of the Parasite

In 1969, two missionary nurses working in a hospital in Lassa, Borno State, Nigeria developed a severe fever with bleeding from various parts of the body. It came on gradually but within a short period both of them had died. At first, the disease was thought to be yellow fever, but subsequent examination found a new virus, a member of the *Arenaviridae* family, to be the cause.

This was a completely new disease, cases had not been reported before, and with its sudden onset, severity and high mortality, it was a considerable worry. Since the original cases occurred, the occasional traveller or expatriate working in West Africa would arrive back in their home country with what appeared to be a flu-like illness, only to rapidly develop severe symptoms similar to those of the two original cases. Lassa fever became established as a new disease, and strict barrier nursing was required to contain it.

However, this did not seem to be the full story, and after some searching it was discovered that Lassa fever, a disease that is highly lethal, especially to persons of non-African origin, was in fact endemic in the community. When the serology had been worked out, people living in the area were found to test positive to the antibody against the disease in their blood. Although the initial cases were found to have been spread from person to person, the pattern of positive serological cases suggested that there was a local animal reservoir of infection. Numerous animals were caught and tested, and eventually the multimammate rat, *Mastomys natalensis*, was incriminated. The rat was particularly troublesome to the villagers as it attacked their grain stores, invariably contaminating them with its urine and faeces while it fed. So it was either eating contaminated grain or inhaling contaminated dust that infected people.

Children probably met the infection first, and as with other childhood infections, such as chickenpox, developed immunity. As well as Nigeria, the endemic area was found to include Sierra Leone, Liberia, Guinea and the Central African Republic. If you came into this area as an adult and acquired the infection, you were liable to get the disease severely, so cases have been reported from the surrounding countries of Mali, Ghana, Côte d'Ivoire and Burkina Faso.

Development of immunity is one of the mechanisms humans have developed to defend themselves from infecting organisms, and Lassa fever illustrates what normally happens when a disease is met for the first time. As a completely new infection (to those from outside the endemic area), people had no inherent defence and developed a severe reaction, which very often led to the death of the individual. If they had experienced the infection as children, when they were developing their library of immune responses, they suffered only mild infection or showed no ill effects. When they met the disease again, their immune system already had experience of the infection and was able to immediately destroy it. Indeed, in many infections, repeated assault by the same organism reactivates the defence mechanism and makes it even stronger.

If this mechanism was to occur through random mutation it would take such a long time that change would not be effective during the person's lifetime, so the B-cells (B-lymphocytes) of the immune mechanism use transposons (jumping genes) to produce the required modification. The cells appear to be able to search for the required gene in their DNA, snip out the piece needed and transfer this to a new site, in effect rewriting the genetic sequence. A tailor-made antibody will then be produced when a person is stressed by the same antigen again. While this process can occur with some antigens during the course of the person's life, it is particularly active during childhood when the antibody library is being built.

The development of immunity becomes such an inherent part of a child's growth that any minor illness that develops is probably no more than a passing inconvenience. However, if that illness develops as an adult, the consequences can be severe. As with Lassa to the non-immune European who is unfortunate enough to meet this disease, the mild infection of chickenpox that most people meet in childhood can be a severe illness to the non-immune adult. It causes respiratory and (particularly) cardiac symptoms, and can lead to damage to the heart. In Pacific Islands where chickenpox was an unknown disease when it was first introduced, it had a devastating effect, and even now in elderly people in these same communities it presents as a cardiomyopathy, producing sudden death.

This pattern of immunity is very characteristic of viral and of most bacterial infections, but with larger organisms a different pattern develops. With the parasitic worms, it is more like an arms race; as they set out to attack the human, the human mounts a defence until a stalemate is gradually reached.

Trichinella spiralis is normally a parasite of pigs, but if humans should inadvertently become infected, normally by eating insufficiently cooked pork, such as in sausages or from a spit-roasted animal, the larval nematode worms are carried to all parts of the body. Here, they are attacked by the body defence mechanisms, resulting in a severe reaction that produces fever, headache and muscle pain, with some people dying from heart or nervous system damage. Once the severe reaction is over, the surviving larvae are encapsulated and cause no further trouble.

Other nematode worms are found in the intestines, and such is the degree of tolerance that has developed between parasite and host that most people do not even know they are infected. *Trichuris trichiura,* the whipworm, is so common (an estimated 795 million are infected) that on routine examination of the stools many people are found to have it. The parasite appears to cause no symptoms and is easily transferred from one person to another, generally through food from contaminated fingers. Only in the young child can the sheer quantity of worms have a debilitating effect. When there are over 16,000 eggs per gram of faeces, a chronic bloody diarrhoea, anaemia and rectal prolapse can result. On its own, or combined with other parasitic infestations that are the lot of the child in developing countries, whipworm infestation can produce sufficient debility to result in the demise of large numbers of children.

Childhood infestation apart, *Trichuris* in the asymptomatic adult illustrates the ultimate status quo of the parasitic worms arms race. With a new infection such as severe acute respiratory syndrome (SARS) or Lassa fever, there is such a severe reaction that a high death rate results, while at the opposite extreme, *Trichuris* produces such little reaction that it can be presumed to be a very old infection of humans. We have become so adapted to it that the parasite can continue its way of life without the host needing to make attempts to get rid of it. Parasitic worms might even confer some advantage, as will be mentioned in Chapter 14.

Evolutionary biologists have trouble with this conclusion and argue that organisms tend to become more virulent. The pathogen needs to disperse its progeny so the more successful it is in upsetting the host defences, such as by causing sneezing or diarrhoea, the greater the number that will be expelled into the environment. Also, infecting organisms are often in competition, e.g. the common cold is produced by many different viruses and at any one time there may be several of them competing with each other to dominate the host. The most virulent will be the most successful because it will be more able to exploit the environmental niche.

However, in both of these arguments there is a limit to virulence, if it is too severe, the host will die and the parasite will fail to spread to other individuals. Also, in a respiratory infection, if the person is prostrated and confined to bed, they will not come in contact with other individuals no matter how much they sneeze or smear surfaces with their droplets. How much more effective in spreading the disease is the host that is a little ill but is still able to move around, contacting other people and contaminating the environment with his/her effusions. This situation will favour a less virulent variant or species that is able to have less effect on its host but produce infective forms, albeit in lesser numbers, for a longer period of time.

There is a similar scenario with gut infections in that the person with severe diarrhoea will be incapacitated, limiting their contamination of the environment, whereas the person with the milder infection will remain ambulatory, and be able to spread the disease. This of course infers that there are poor or absent means of disposing of faeces and that handwashing is not carried out. Indeed, taken to its logical conclusions, as with *T. trichiura*, there is no need to stimulate the host to have diarrhoea at all. Diarrhoea will produce an increase in the number of eggs shed to the environment for a short period, but just normal stool output will produce a regular dispersal of eggs over a very long period, possibly the full lifespan of the host. If this is combined with no handwashing, many more people will be infected in total.

The ultimate stage of decreased virulence is the development of vaccines, as discussed below.

A further argument in favour of a tendency for increasing virulence is the speed with which bacteria and viruses are able to mutate, meaning that there is a greater chance of more virulent variants being produced. This has indeed happened, e.g. with influenza, but then the epidemic pattern of an infectious disease comes into play (Fig. 3.1).

When an infectious disease starts there will be a population of susceptible individuals, generally in close contact with each other, so the infection will rapidly spread to reach a peak, after which it decreases. This is because people will either die from the disease or recover from it and become immune, thus decreasing the number of susceptibles in the population. Providing that more susceptible people do not enter the population, the disease will eventually die out. At the same time as this is happening, the immune mechanism of those who have recovered has modified its immune response so should that variant of the organism return they will be protected.

Evolutionary theory suggests that diseases spread by arthropod vectors (mosquitoes, fleas, lice, etc.) will favour more virulent forms. This is seen in tropical Africa, where although all species of *Plasmodium* are present, the most virulent, *P. falciparum*, predominates. This virulence is due to the parasite invading more red blood cells than *P. vivax* or the other two human species of malaria, thereby causing more destruction and an increased production of parasites, and facilitating greater transmission.

This theory shows that it is in the interests of the parasite to cause the least harm to its vector but to immobilize the host. If the person contracting malaria is made so ill that they remain inactive and prostrate,

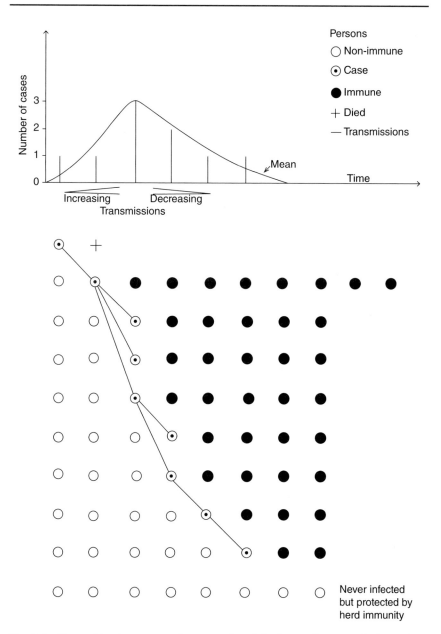

Fig. 3.1. The epidemic curve and course of an infection as it proceeds through a limited population (simplified).

allowing mosquitoes to feed on them without being swotted, this will make it easier for the infection to be transmitted.

While *P. falciparum* dominates in Africa, in the more temperate parts of the world where lower temperatures make mosquito survival difficult, or the vector is inefficient, as in much of the Indian subcontinent, then the more persistent but less virulent species *P. vivax* is more commonly found. This parasite has obtained an advantage over *P. falciparum* and the other malaria parasites in being able to complete its development cycle at a lower temperature. At temperatures of 30°C, *P. falciparum* takes 9 days to complete its life cycle, while at 19°C it takes in excess of 30 days, longer than the life expectancy of the average mosquito. In contrast, *P. vivax* can complete its developmental cycle in 20 days at this lower temperature, meaning that viable transmission can still take place.

In malaria, as the number of developmental forms in the mosquito (called oocysts) increases, so their survival decreases, while in filariasis (Chapter 4), heavy infection with microfilariae will lead to the death of the mosquito. Similarly, the plague-carrying flea is killed by the parasite blocking its feeding apparatus, and the louse in epidemic typhus is generally crushed in the process of transferring infection. There seem to be just as many exceptions to evolutionary theory, and to so-called 'Evolutionary or Darwinian Medicine' (as proposed by Nesse and Williams in 1994).

The problem is that evolutionary theory is based on non-human animals, mainly looking at one side of the equation – the selection of the parasite to attack the host. The other aspect is the response of the host to the infection (and it is much more difficult to measure the host response in animals). Initially, host response is the most severe, but it decreases in severity as the virulence of the parasite also decreases. In other words, it is a matched response leading to a compromise, or the evolutionary tendency applied to the parasite is countered by the same evolutionary response of the host. A balance is achieved, as with much of nature. (Host response is further discussed below.)

Malaria as a Complex Disease

The major cause of death in children in Africa is malaria, where not only does *P. falciparum* predominate, but the most efficient mosquito, *Anopheles gambiae*, is also present. This combination results in almost constant infection.

The young child in the malaria endemic area of Africa probably fights the greatest battle that it will ever have to fight in these first few years of its life. When it is inoculated with malaria parasites it will develop fever and have its first attack of malaria, from which it will either die or survive. It is not able to develop absolute immunity as it would to viral infections, but depends upon repeated infection right through until adult life. The centre of this immunity-producing mechanism and also of the red blood cells that are being destroyed by the malaria is the spleen, which increases in size to such an extent that it distends the abdomen. This enlargement of the spleen is so marked that it can be used as a measure of malaria endemicity. The greatest degree of endemicity, called *holoendemi-city*, is a spleen rate (the number of enlarged spleens per 100 similar aged individuals) in children of constantly over 75%.

Approximately 1 million children used to die each year from malaria, but this has been reduced to some 600,000 annually in the last decade owing to the use of insecticide-treated mosquito nets (ITNs) and other interventions. The treated mosquito net is a very simple improvement on an old strategy to provide a barrier between the sleeping person and the mosquito. Impregnating the material with insecticide not only enhances this barrier but kills any mosquitoes that come in contact with the net.

Once the child survives the initial attack of malaria and builds up its immunity, it becomes ambulatory, depriving mosquitoes of the ease of taking a blood meal that there would be if the person had been prostrate. It can, therefore, be hypothesized that the use of mosquito nets will select for less virulent strains of malaria because the interval between mosquito biting will be extended and there will be advantage to a parasite adaptation to an ambulatory person. This has indeed been seen to happen in Solomon Islands where an extensive programme of providing mosquito nets has been in operation. Formerly, most of the cases of malaria were *P. falciparum*, now they are nearly all *P. vivax*.

This situation can be complicated by the mosquito changing its habits, as happened with the use of residual insecticides in the malaria eradication programmes. When this was the strategy, in one programme the mosquito changed its biting habit from being a night-time biter, reaching a peak around midnight, to one of dawn and dusk biting. This was when people got up to work in the fields and when they returned in the evening, so were no longer protected by insecticides sprayed in their houses. Although mosquitoes are not pathogens themselves, they, like all of nature, have to adapt to survive.

When the child becomes an adult it is immune to malaria, providing it continues to have repeated challenge from malaria parasites, but if the adult leaves the endemic area for any long period of time then its immunity will diminish and it becomes susceptible again. This has been the tragic result of several brilliant Africans that have gone to Europe or North America for further studies, where they lose their immunity, so that when they return and do not take precautions, they succumb to severe malaria. This is also a problem for the pregnant woman, especially in her first pregnancy, as the body reduces its immune response during pregnancy, and in so doing makes her more susceptible to malaria, requiring her to be protected during this period.

By what must be one of the most unexpected occurrences in nature is where one disease produces protection against another. A chance mutation in sub-Saharan Africans resulted in sickle cell disease, in which during a sickling crisis, the red blood cells take on abnormal shapes and the person suffers from severe anaemia or dies. However, the mutation can be carried quite passively if it is inherited from only one parent, so that the individual is heterozygous, and this confers protection from getting severe malaria. Sickle cell disease would normally have been expected to have died out or become very rare, but because of its protective effect on malaria, 40% of people carry the sickle-cell gene in the malarial parts of Africa.

The malaria parasite needs to enter the red blood cell to reproduce asexually and evolution has come up with a number of strategies over the millions of years that it has been tested by this parasite. The Duffy blood group favours parasite entry by allowing the parasite to stick to the red blood cell, but many people in West Africa carry a Duffy-minus mutation, which gives them protection. In the Mediterranean, there are people with whole sections of the haemoglobin molecule that have been deleted; this protects by slowing the growth of *Plasmodium*, but those with this mutation suffer from thalassaemia (the anaemia of the sea). Fortunately, malaria is rare now in the Mediterranean, so there is no advantage in this mutation and over time it will be selected against.

Stephen Oppenheimer, while investigating anaemia in children in Papua New Guinea, found that alpha thalassaemia was the cause but, as with the disease in the Mediterranean, thalassaemia had a protective effect on contracting malaria. This started off his interest in human genetics, and he has since become a leading authority in the origins of humans, sampling genetic patterns from many different peoples in the world.

One of these protecting factors was only discovered because of an unexpected reaction to drugs. During the Korean War, some American soldiers of African descent became anaemic when treated with primaquine. Ironically, primaquine is used to treat chronic malaria as it removes the liver stage in *P. vivax* infection, but it causes a reaction in people that lack glucose-6-phosphate-dehydrogenase, or G6PD deficiency for short. It later transpired that the reason people of African descent had this susceptibility was that G6PD deficiency, like the other mechanisms just described, makes the red blood cell less suitable to parasitization by *Plasmodium*.

As well as their reaction to primaquine and some other medicaments, people with G6PD deficiency had a similar experience when they ate broad beans, which are more widely known as the fava bean (from the Italian). This resulted in a haemolytic anaemia that could be fatal. So like sickle cell anaemia, a potential fatal mutation was maintained in the population because it protected against malaria.

The gene for G6PD deficiency is carried on the X-chromosome, so in the male there is some protection, but in the female, with two X-chromosomes, not only is there a greater chance that she will have this protective effect on at least one of her chromosomes, but also the possibility that it might be on both, doubly enhancing the effect. This is particularly relevant to the pregnant woman, as her immune status is lowered during pregnancy, so G6PD deficiency protects her during this period. It is even more important as an evolutionary mechanism, because it means that having this trait protects her in the production of more offspring. So natural selection has determined this condition to continue, despite the dangers of adverse reaction to the fava bean and, more recently, to certain drugs.

Amphibiosis

Another unexpected paradox is where a disease-producing organism becomes protective for some of the time; this is given the name of amphibiosis. The most unusual of parasites (because it lives in the mucus-covered lining of the very hostile environment produced by stomach acid), *Helicobacter pylori*, was incriminated in the pathology of stomach ulcers and, more seriously, stomach cancer. These are still major concerns, but *H. pylori* has also been found to be protective against acid reflux of the lower end of the oesophagus, which, in turn, can lead to cancer of this part of the body. If you have *H. pylori*, you are at increased risk of getting stomach cancer; if you don't have it, you are at increased risk of cancer of the oesophagus. There are few more unusual conundrums.

On balance though, it seems that having *H. pylori* in early life is beneficial and that the increased use of antibiotics in children has removed its protective effect. Strange as it may seem, this bacterium appears to play a vital role in damping down allergic reactions and may be the reason why children treated with antibiotics early in life are more prone to develop asthma and other allergic disorders, as discussed more fully in Chapter 14.

Host Response

While the disappearance of *H. pylori* in developed and other countries that use considerable amounts of antibiotics (led by China, which now has the highest rate of antibiotic use of any country), this is not the situation in most developing countries, where clinics often run out of treatment or parents are not able to take their children the long distance required to get help. This is particularly the case with lower respiratory infections, which includes the condition we commonly know as pneumonia. What starts off as a trivial respiratory infection may develop into a life-threatening one, probably made worse by the child's nutritional state. This is another factor in the host/parasite relationship that is often forgotten: the state of the host.

It is common practice to tag microorganisms with their degree of virulence, as though a particular organism will be more lethal than another, but just as important, in fact more so with respiratory infections, is the status of the host. Some people readily contract tuberculosis, while others do not, and in children, an infecting organism that causes a mild respiratory infection in one will produce a serious illness in the next. This might be due to the nutritional status of the child, or to it having another minor illness, but often it is in the inherent genetic make-up of the individual.

While the overuse of antibiotics is possibly leading to increased rates of asthma in developing countries (see Chapter 14), their non-use in developing countries is leading to high rates of death from respiratory infections. It is necessary to be speedy in starting treatment for a severe respiratory infection, and considerable emphasis is placed on trying to get children to be brought early, so that their minor respiratory infection does not turn into their death sentence.

Lower respiratory infections are the commonest cause of ill health and death from communicable disease in the world. In 2012, there were 3.1 million deaths from non-tuberculosis disease and 0.9 million from tuberculosis, making the combined deaths from respiratory disease by far the most important type of disease process. Second to respiratory infections were diarrhoeal diseases, here again predominantly infecting children, with 1.5 million deaths. The major cause of diarrhoeal disease is poor water supplies, a problem mentioned many times in the following pages.

The host response is an important component of the body defence mechanisms in most illnesses, though to varying degrees. In response to the brute force of *T. spiralis*, boring its way into the body, the host response immobilizes and localizes the parasite. In viral and bacterial infections, the immune system is normally sufficient on its own, especially if it has been stimulated by having previously met antigens from the organism and generated antibodies to them. Some of the larger parasites, such as the roundworm *Ascaris*, are able to secrete a protective layer that hides them from attack by the immune system of the intestines. Going down a scale in size are the trypanosomes of sleeping sickness, which are able to frequently change their form and so evade the immune system in this way. The HIV virus continually mutates so that as soon as the body has learnt the antibody characteristics of the virus, the virus has changed, thus exhausting the host's ability to produce immune complexes.

Surprisingly, the HIV virus, despite its short contact with human beings, finds its passage into cells of the body facilitated by the presence of the enzyme reverse transcriptase. This is not required at all by its host, so it seems strange we should have a protein that not only do we not require but that aids infection with retroviruses. It transpires that much of the human genome contains non-coding or junk DNA, which has no apparent purpose in our continued existence, but that some of it, like the gene for reverse transcriptase, has been put there by previous retroviruses. A disease has actually implanted its own disease-facilitating gene into our genome!

Human Endogenous Retroviruses

In looking in more detail into non-coding DNA, scientists have found that some 50% of it was put there by jumping genes. Similar to the gene for reverse transcriptase, and inserted by an unknown retrovirus, some jumping genes (retrotransposons) might even be retroviruses themselves. In other words, a part of the human genome has been hijacked by viruses, and as in the development of the eukaryotic cell described in Chapter 1, a disease-producing particle (in this case a virus) has actually been able to manipulate our DNA.

Retroviruses carry out their reverse synthesizing ability by converting RNA into DNA, instead of the other way round, which is the usual process. Cells use their DNA to instruct RNA to produce new cells from proteins, but retroviruses, which are made of RNA, use reverse transcriptase to change their RNA into DNA. Now with DNA, they have the ability to alter the genetic code, which seems to be how some of the non-coding DNA was produced.

So far, at least 8% of the human genome has been identified as being retroviruses, now called human endogenous retroviruses or HERVs. Although they may have set out with the intention of manipulating the human genome for their own use, any negative modification would have been eliminated by natural selection. But like the mitochondria of the human cell that arose by conversion from a bacterium to our benefit, so are most of the HERVs that have so far been identified to our benefit, most likely because of their capacity to produce mutations.

Bacteria can mutate much faster than we can, such as coming up with a resistance gene to an antibiotic, but viruses can mutate even faster, which we could have used to our benefit. Useful mutations can be found at a much greater rate in this way, and may have led to our rapid evolution at the expense of other animals. A suggestion that this is indeed what happened is the surprisingly high number of HERVs on the X- and Y-chromosomes, particularly the latter. Half of all the genes on the Y-chromosome are retroposon-like, which is a significantly greater number than are found on the chimpanzee genome. This would suggest that they may be the 'Holy Grail' that makes us human. Could it be that such attributes as speech, language, learning and reasoning were put there by these HERVs? If this is the case, then it would indicate that we are even more directed by viruses than we could ever have possibly conceived could be the case.

The action of several of the HERVs seems quite diverse compared with what must have been their original function, because six have been shown to be necessary in the formation of the placenta, while others were involved in the development of the brain, as mentioned in Chapter 2.

Manipulation of the host by parasites is a very ancient strategy and although we only have one human example in toxoplasmosis (Chapter 11), it might well be that we have inherited this ability from our ancestral line as a result of infection by viruses millions of years ago. One of the most successful of all parasitic insects is the endoparasitic wasp. This has the very unpleasant habit of injecting its eggs directly into prey species, which then hatch and eat their way out, feeding on the tissues of the unfortunate victim. In order to facilitate this process, viral infection stimulates the wasp to also inject teratocyte cells, which are trophic and immunosuppressive, and manipulate the host's endocrine system to favour the developing embryo. These trophic and immunosuppressive functions are needed in the development of the mammalian placenta, which helps to explain how the HERVs that we have inherited might be involved in this process. To the mother, the developing fetus is recognized as a parasite, so parasite defence mechanisms, suppression of the mother's immune mechanisms and a trophic-seeking tissue that forms the placenta are required. These appear to have come originally from the virus infecting the endoparasitic wasp that was in our distant ancestry.

It will be intriguing to know what other remarkable revelations will arise as more of our HERVs, and perhaps other parts of the junk DNA, are sequenced, such that we might have to conclude that not only have viruses been manipulating us for a considerable period of time, but that we have benefited from the many ingenious methods that natural selection has given parasites. We may even be more parasite than non-parasite!

This all seems a difficult concept to grapple with while the human race is being ravaged by the most destructive retrovirus we have ever met: HIV. However, there is already a suggestion that HIV is changing its virulence, as was outlined in the BBC News of 1 December 2014, based on an interview with Professor Philip Goulder, part of a research team (mainly) from Oxford University (Payne and Muenchhoff *et al.*, 2014). Such is the speed of viral replication that this team showed that HIV is already evolving into a less infective form. When HIV attacks someone with a particularly effective immune mechanism, the virus has to change in order to survive, by reducing its ability to replicate, which means that the rate of transmission from person to person will be prolonged. This appears to have happened in Botswana, which has a longer history of the disease than does South Africa, where the infection was introduced a decade later. The researchers found that there was already a 10% lower replication rate in the older HIV in Botswana than in the newer form in South Africa.

Also mentioned in the report of this research was the suggestion that antiretroviral therapy (ART) primarily attacks the more virulent strains of the virus, allowing milder forms to survive. Some 20 years ago, the interval between infection and the development of acquired immune deficiency syndrome (AIDS) was on average 10 years, while in Botswana this has now been prolonged to 12.5 years. So in time, like some of the other infections described above, one can anticipate that HIV will become a mild infection in humans, as it was in its original chimpanzee host.

Unfortunately, it has already developed resistance to several of the drugs used in ART, so like another arms race – that between bacteria and the development of antibiotics (discussed in Chapter 19), new drugs will need to be found if this scenario is to occur.

Vaccination

With a disease that has never been met before, such as SARS, the initial reaction is severe, with a high mortality rate. As more people became infected and the disease-producing organism is passaged (passed) through further individuals, its potency normally decreases. This happens with a number of organisms, particularly the viruses, and is the principle underlying the production of vaccines.

Utilizing a susceptible but non-human subject (such as a mouse or guinea pig) the virus that is used to infect a batch of animals is recovered and given to another batch of animals. This process is repeated many times until the organism has only its antibody-stimulating ability, and will not cause illness. Vaccines have been produced from attenuated organisms (living organisms that have had their potency reduced to harmlessness), dead organisms, toxins or components of organisms, and they are one of the greatest advances made to protect people against disease-producing organisms.

As well as protecting the individual, if given to a sufficient number of people, a vaccine will also protect those that have missed being vaccinated, an effect that is known as herd immunity. In a limited population, as infection proceeds, fewer and fewer susceptible people will remain, until there is an insufficient number to allow continued transmission. A few people will escape becoming infected because of the decreasing chance that they will contact an infected individual (see Fig. 3.1). The same principle can be used with a vaccination programme, so that varying with the infectiousness of the organism, only some 85% to 90% of the population needs to be vaccinated. The problem is that new people are entering this population as immigrants or, more commonly, as newborns, so they need to be vaccinated to keep the herd immunity sufficiently high. If this is not done, then after a few years there will be sufficient non-immunized individuals to allow transmission to take place again. Unfortunately, this was seen with measles outbreaks that occurred as a result of misinformed parents refusing to have their children vaccinated, sometimes with tragic results. There is a similar danger with rubella (German measles) vaccination.

The rubella vaccine protects the pregnant woman from developing infection in the early part of pregnancy, which is when it will cause severe damage to her fetus. Two strategies can be used: either give the vaccine to adolescent girls, so that they will be protected when they become pregnant, in which case the virus will always be present in the community (as there will be sufficient susceptible males); or give the vaccine to both males and females of adolescent age, with the objective of eliminating rubella from the population. Clearly, the latter would be the more desirable policy, though if the level of vaccination is insufficient, there will be enough non-immune people in the community to allow an outbreak, which will infect females when they are older and possibly pregnant. It is, therefore, vital that once a policy of eliminating rubella from the community is embarked upon, that a high level of vaccination is maintained.

In 2013, just this problem occurred in Japan when there was an outbreak of 5442 cases of rubella. Although three-quarters of these were in males, the occurrence of the disease indicated that the eradication policy was not working. Furthermore, several of these cases travelled to other countries, thus stressing the need for high levels of immunization to be maintained.

A Balance between Nature and Disease

Vaccination is a method of increasing our immune response and protecting us from disease, but for some vaccines, it is only effective when maternal antibodies that are produced by the mother to protect the newborn infant are no longer present. Vaccines are most suitably given at certain ages to produce the best response, and there are dangers in giving them to some people, such as those with HIV infection, who may develop adverse reactions. Immunity has been a valuable mechanism for protecting us against disease but it also poses problems for the body, particularly during pregnancy.

The objective of natural selection is to pass on genetic material to the next generation so as to maintain the species, in other words to encourage reproduction and the development of offspring. In the face of constant attack by disease organisms, immune mechanisms were developed, but the fetus is identified as a foreign organism with a tendency by the mother's body to reject it. In order to overcome this danger, two protective mechanisms come into play, the immune status of the mother is lowered during pregnancy and the placental barrier prevents a mixing of the blood of the mother and the fetus. Natural selection and disease selection are in opposition to each other and in this situation a balance has developed between them.

Using a Vector

4

It is natural to think that parasites are setting out to attack humans and cause illness, but life is a competition, and all life forms, including parasites, are seeking to derive benefit for themselves by living off other animals. Many of the infections that afflict us have very simple means of transmission – through poor hygiene, so that organisms on our fingers are swallowed, leading to diarrhoeal disease, or from coughing, during which clouds of organisms are cast into the surrounding air to infect people that are close by. Other organisms have developed more complex life cycles and, at certain stages, depend on an intermediate organism – a vector – to carry the infective form to the host.

Anopheline Mosquitoes

It was Patrick Manson (1844–1922), a Scottish doctor who had gone to China at the suggestion of his brother, who worked out the life cycle of filariasis in 1877. His gardener, Hin Lo, had an enlarged leg produced by filariasis. Manson found that larvae were present in Hin Lo's blood during the night but not during the day, so he hypothesised that the infection might be transmitted by mosquitoes. He caught the mosquitoes that fed on Hin Lo while he slept, and then dissected them. He later wrote:

> I shall not easily forget the first mosquito I dissected. I tore off its abdomen and succeeded in expressing the blood the stomach contained. Placing this under the microscope I was gratified to find that, so far from killing the Filaria, the digestive juices of the mosquito seemed to have stimulated it to fresh activity.

Manson is regarded as the father of tropical medicine, and on his return to England was instrumental in founding the London School of Tropical Medicine (later the London School of Hygiene and Tropical Medicine). He was a great friend of Ronald Ross (1857–1932), and suggested to Ross the mosquito-transmission theory for malaria.

© R. Webber 2015. *Disease Selection: The Way Disease Changed the World* (R. Webber)

Ross was born in India, the son of an army general, and after training at St Bartholomew's Hospital in London, he joined the Indian Medical Service, determined to look for the way that malaria was transmitted. Although malarious, the mosquitoes responsible for the transmission of malaria in India are not as efficient as those in Africa, so it was not until 1897, after years of effort, that Ross finally saw the developmental stages of the malaria parasite within the *Anopheles* mosquito. He then experimented with bird malaria to work out the reproductive cycle of the malaria parasite, including the development of the infective form within the salivary glands. After he had joined the staff of the Liverpool School of Tropical Medicine, he was sent to West Africa, where he discovered *A. gambiae* to be the main vector of malaria in Africa.

The Nobel Prize had recently been established, and after reading about it Ross put himself forward for the award, which he was justifiably given. One can imagine the negative comments that one would receive if one were to do such a thing today, but as he was working in India and publishing his work in the *Journal of the Indian Medical Service*, it would otherwise probably not have been noticed by the Nobel Committee. As it is, his Nobel Prize was claimed by three countries, India, where Ross was born (and has a fine display in the museum in Kolkata), the UK, of which he was a citizen, and Scotland, from where his ancestral roots originated.

It is surprising that the fragile mosquito, so easily blown by the wind, affected by the light of the moon, and swotted with ease, should be such an important vector of disease. While its place in the transmission of malaria is well known, and perhaps less so its role in filariasis, it is actually the most prevalent vector of disease in the world. At the last count, there were 77 diseases transmitted by mosquitoes, meaning that not only is the mosquito the most important vector of disease, but also that it is responsible for transmitting more diseases than any other means.

The mosquito is found from the Arctic to the equator, as well as ancestral forms having been discovered imprisoned in amber, so it is impossible to work out where it originated. However, the *Anopheles* mosquito has been associated with malaria for a considerable period of time (see Chapter 2), so it is likely that it became a vector of malaria in Africa. *Anopheles* mosquitoes are now found throughout the tropical areas of the world and, when it is warm enough, in suitable habitats outside this region. The number of *Anopheles* species responsible for the transmission of malaria are many, but of these, only some 25 are main vectors.

Alfred Russel Wallace, while collecting specimens in what is now Indonesia, and also realizing the importance of natural selection, noticed that many species of animals progressed no further east than the larger islands of Indonesia. He drew a line to show this demarcation, since called Wallace's line. The line passes between Borneo and Sulawesi, and further south between Bali and Lombok. It was later modified by Max Carl Wilhelm Weber as Weber's Line, which puts this demarcation further east, running between Halmahera and Sulawesi, and skirting round Timor. Interestingly, the *Anopheles* mosquito is also demarcated by another hypothetical line lying still further east, which was mapped by Professor Patrick Buxton of the London School of Hygiene and Tropical Medicine, and is known as Buxton's line. This line runs to the east of New Guinea and the other Melanesian Islands (Solomon Islands, Vanuatu, etc.), and the *Anopheles* mosquito is not found in the many islands of Polynesia (to the east) and Micronesia (to the north); hence, they are free of malaria. Buxton's line does not determine the geographical distribution of other mosquito species, which are extensively found in these islands, bringing with them the scourge of filariasis or devastating epidemics of dengue.

As mentioned in Chapter 8, it was easy for mosquitoes to stow away on slave ships and carry malaria to South America, so it is strange why the same thing did not happen in the dark recesses of the ocean-going canoes that carried the ancestral Polynesians and Micronesians. These peoples originated from or passed through the malarious islands of Melanesia on their way to the many islands of the Pacific, which they subsequently colonized. If the transport of mosquitoes did not happen then, there is every reason to believe that it must have happened several times since, so it seems that *Anopheles* mosquitoes were just unable to adapt and flourish in these small islands.

Of course, Buxton's line also passes between Australia and New Zealand, and many people do not realize that there are the same species of *Anopheles* in the tropical areas of Australia as transmit malaria in New Guinea and the other islands of Melanesia. It was only by conscientious efforts, largely those of Professor Black and his team, that the malaria parasite was eradicated from the vast area of northern Australia. The *Anopheles* mosquito itself was not eradicated though, and still feeds upon anyone that should expose their flesh to these insects during the evening sundowner.

Culicine Mosquitoes

Of the other 75 infections transmitted by mosquitoes, all are viral diseases (see Table 4.1 for the main ones of importance). What is surprising is that they are nearly all transmitted by the other great family of mosquitoes, the culicines (*Culex* and *Aedes* genera), the anophelines (*Anopheles*) having become so specialized that they only transmit malaria, filariasis and two of the arboviral (**ar**thropod **bo**rne **vir**al) infections.

Many of the arbovirus infections present with encephalitis, infection of the brain, which seems difficult to explain as mosquitoes produce infection when taking a blood meal, yet the brain is surrounded by membranes that make what is called the blood–brain barrier. Most infections that enter the blood do not affect the brain unless they find a way of crossing this

Table 4.1. The important arboviral infections of humans. (From Webber, 2012, *Communicable Diseases: A Global Perspective*, 4th Edn.)

Virus	Distribution	Vectors	Reservoir
Mainly fever or arthritis			
Chikungunya	Africa, South and South-east Asia	*Aedes (Ae.) aegypti, Ae.africanus, Ae. albopictus*	Baboons, bats, rodents, monkeys
O'nyong-nyong	East Africa, Senegal	*Anopheles (A.) gambiae, A. funestus*	Mosquitoes?
West Nile	Africa, Asia, Europe, USA	*Culex pipens molestus, C. modestus, C. univittatus*	Birds
Oropuche	Trinidad, South America	Mosquitoes, possibly *Culicoides*	Monkeys, sloths, birds
Orungo	West Africa, Uganda	*Ae. dentatus, Anopheles* spp.	Humans?
Ross River	Australia, New Zealand, Pacific Islands	*C. annulirostris, Ae. vigilax, Ae. polynesiensis*	Mosquitoes
Fever and encephalitis			
Western equine	Americas	*C. tarsalis, Culiseta (Cs.) melanura*	Birds
Eastern equine	Americas, Caribbean	*Cs. melanura, Aedes* and *Coquillettidia* spp.	Birds, rodents
St Louis	Americas, Caribbean	*C. tarsalis, C. nigripalpus, C. quinquefasciatus*	Birds
Venezuelan equine	Central/South America, Caribbean, parts of USA	*C. tarsalis* and other *Culex, Aedes, Mansonia, Sabethes, Psorophora, Anopheles, Haemagogus* spp.	Rodents
Japanese	East, South and South-east Asia	*C. tritaeniorhynchus, C. gelidus, C. fuscocephala*	Birds, pigs
Murray Valley	New Guinea, Australia	*C. annulirostris*	Birds
Rocio	Brazil	Probably mosquitoes	Birds? Rodents
Haemorrhagic fevers			
Yellow fever	South America and Africa	*Ae. aegypti, Ae. africanus, Ae. simpsoni, Ae. furcifer/taylori, Ae. luteocephalus, Haemagogus* spp.	Monkeys, mosquitoes
Dengue 1, 2, 3 and 4	Asia, Pacific, Caribbean, Africa, Americas	*Ae. aegypti, Ae. albopictus, Ae. scutellaris* group, *Ae. niveus, Ochlerotatus*	Human/ Mosquito, (monkeys in jungle cycle)

Continued

Table 4.1. Continued.

Virus	Distribution	Vectors	Reservoir
Rift Valley	Africa, South-west Asia	*Ae. caballus, C. theileri, C. quinquefasciatus* and other *Culex* and *Aedes* spp.	Sheep, cattle, etc., mosquitoes
Kyasanur Forest	South India	*Haemaphysalis* (hard ticks)	Rodents, monkeys
Crimean–Congo	Europe, Africa, Asia	*Hyalomma* spp. (hard ticks)	Domestic animals

blood–brain barrier. However, there is another route, along the nerves themselves, which avoids the immune cells of the blood that are always ready to disarm infective agents, and this would seem to be the way many arboviruses successfully attack humans. (The rabies virus is another and better known example of a cause of viral encephalitis.)

Many of the culicine mosquitoes are particularly opportunistic, most people probably having been bitten by the incongruously named *Culex quinquefasciatus*, the common daytime-biting mosquito that is found in so many parts of the world. (It used to be called *Culex pipiens fatigans*, or just *C. fatigans*, a much more manageable name, but somebody discovered that it had been originally given the longer name and so by the convention of precedence we are lumbered with this mouthful every time we want to talk about it.) It particularly likes to breed in polluted water, such as that found in blocked drains, and somehow finds its way into your hotel room in most tropical cities.

Another culicine mosquito, and an important vector of virus diseases, is the *Aedes* group of mosquitoes. These are one of the few mosquitoes that can be identified with the naked eye owing to their distinctive black and white colouring (see Fig. 4.1). *Ae. aegypti* is the main vector of the dengue and yellow fever viruses, while *Ae. albopictus* has recently invaded North America, where it was responsible for an outbreak of West Nile virus that resulted in 3231 cases and 176 deaths in the USA, as well as many more in Canada. The *Aedes* mosquito will readily breed in any collections of water, such as old tins, coconut shells, water tanks or one of their favourite places, old tyres. These collect water really easily, and it is extremely difficult to remove unless holes are cut in the tyres; it is thought that it was the trade in used tyres that introduced *Ae. albopictus* to North America, where it has now taken up permanent residence.

As well as the West Nile virus infecting humans, it has also caused a high mortality in crows in the eastern USA. The virus does not appear to persist in wild birds, but because they exist in large flocks there may be sufficient numbers to permit a chain of transmission and so serve as a temporary reservoir.

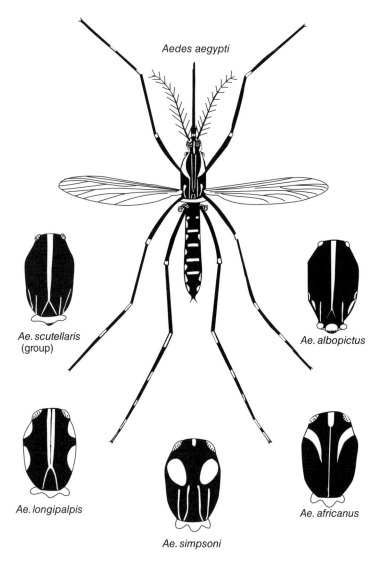

Fig. 4.1. The black and white mosquitoes, *Aedes*. (From Webber, 2012, *Communicable Diseases: A Global Perspective*, 4th Edn.)

We have little evidence that arboviral infections cause much harm to the mosquito, while with malaria, any harm to the mosquito is proportional to the number of parasites. But with another vector-transmitted disease, filariasis, the mosquito is killed by heavy infections of the parasite; it was the comparatively large size of the infecting organism that allowed Patrick Manson to identify it, and this is what causes the problem for the mosquito.

Filariasis and Its Control

In 2010, there were estimated to be 1.39 billion people – some 18% of the world population – at risk of developing filariasis in 72 countries and territories, yet apart from its gross manifestations of elephantiasis (permanent disfiguring enlargement of the legs, breasts and scrotum), few people know much about it. Some 120 million people are infected with this disease, and at least 40 million of these have the disabling form. The main reason for this is that filariasis does not kill, but to be disabled with it is a life sentence as there is no effective cure for elephantiasis.

The infecting organism is a nematode worm, the larval stage of which is carried by mosquitoes – both anopheline and culicine. The larvae escape on to the skin of the person bitten when the mosquito takes a blood meal, and from here they find their way into the body, generally through the bite site and to the lymphatics. In the body, the larvae are carried in the lymph to a regional lymph node where they develop into adults. Both male and female worms must meet to produce larvae, which are then taken up from a blood vessel when another mosquito comes to feed (see Fig. 4.2). This is one of the most complex life cycles of any parasite, as not only is a vector involved (in which development takes place) but both adult male and female worms must find each other for larvae (microfilariae) to be produced at the optimum time for them to be taken up by a mosquito. This is during the night-time hours if the main vector is an *Anopheles* mosquito – the pattern in Africa, or during the daytime if it is a *Culex* mosquito – as found in India. Take-up is by both day and night by the vector *Aedes* mosquito in the pattern in Polynesian Pacific Islands, yet the parasite has developed differing peak periods for its larvae (known as periodicity) to coincide with each of these three mosquito vectors.

Although the nematode larva is microscopic, it is a comparatively big organism for the fragile mosquito to accommodate. After the larva has been taken up into the mosquito's stomach during its blood meal on a human, it bores its way into the thoracic muscles where two of its developmental stages take place, which limits the flying ability of the mosquito. If the number of larvae ingested by the mosquito are too many, then they will kill the mosquito, as shown in Fig. 4.3. (point E), which is a mathematical representation of the level of filariasis infection related to the number of parasites, for the two main types of mosquitoes, culicine (*Culex* and *Aedes*) and anopheline. The line P represents proportionality, so that above it, infection will take place, and below it, infection will die out. This shows that for the culicine pattern of transmission (top), the more larvae (microfilariae) ingested, the greater the increase in the rate of infection, up to point E, where mosquito mortality takes place and transmission becomes unsustained. With anopheline transmission, the graph is similar, but there is in addition a lower point (I), below which transmission does not take place. This is due to the anopheline mosquito having a pharyngeal

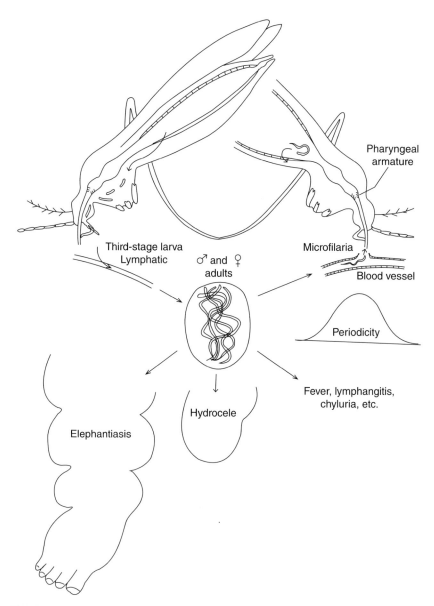

Fig. 4.2. The life cycle and clinical features of lymphatic filariasis. (From Webber, 2012, *Communicable Diseases: A Global Perspective*, 4th Edn.)

armature, which is rather like a set of teeth that damage the microfilariae when they are ingested. This means that in low levels of human infection, transmission does not take place, because there are only a few damaged microfilariae taken up by the mosquito when it takes a blood meal. However, after a certain level of infection is reached, there are sufficient

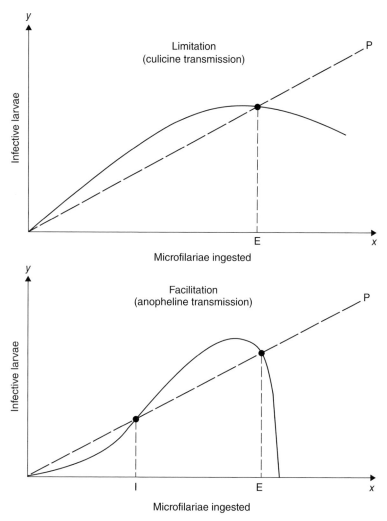

Fig. 4.3 The dynamics of culicine and anopheline transmitted filariasis. (Reproduced by permission, from Pichon, G., Perrault, G. and Laigret J. (1975) *Rendement parasitaire chez les vecteurs de filarioses.* (WHO/FIL/75.132), World Health Organization, Geneva.)

microfilariae taken up for some of them to be ingested undamaged, hence transmission increases. This continues until the number of ingested and surviving larvae causes mosquito mortality, and the infection cannot be sustained.

The pattern of infection just described has implications for control whereby reducing the level of parasites in humans to below point I for anopheline mosquitoes means that the disease will die out. This can either be done by using drugs that kill the microfilariae, which means treating a sufficient proportion of the population, or by reducing the number of mosquitoes, so that less than the threshold number of parasites (I) is transmitted. The threshold number of parasites was worked out in China and was also measured for a species of *Anopheles* mosquito in Solomon Islands. (It should also be noted that as the level of transmission for culicine mosquitoes starts from zero, control needs to be virtually perfect.)

The problem here is that if just drugs are used to kill the microfilariae then the number of larvae ingested by the mosquito is reduced and the mosquito is helped to be fitter and live longer. If this mosquito is an *Anopheles* mosquito that also transmits malaria – the situation in much of Africa and the Melanesian part of the Pacific – then by producing healthier mosquitoes the ability of these mosquitoes to transmit malaria is increased. This means that the preferable strategy is to control the mosquitoes, such as with the use of insecticide-treated mosquito nets (ITNs); if drug treatment is used for the disease, then mosquito control must be practised as well. Indeed, this is one of the few examples where one control method, the use of ITNs, can control two diseases, malaria and filariasis, at the same time.

Uniquely, it is with filariasis that there is another example of one treatment being an effective control strategy for more than one disease, in that one of the drugs used to reduce the number of microfilariae, albendazole, is also effective in treating intestinal parasites, especially *Trichuris*, *Ascaris* (roundworms) and hookworms. As it is given in a mass treatment programme for filariasis, this is a similar strategy to that used by the Rockefeller Foundation in controlling hookworm infection, mentioned in Chapter 7.

The Tsetse Fly and Sleeping Sickness

What would seem to be a much more likely vector than the fragile mosquito, because it is a strong flier and a sturdier built insect, is the tsetse fly, the vector of sleeping sickness in Africa. The tsetse fly has one of the most painful bites of any insect and will descend in vast numbers to bite you even through your clothes, should you be passing through its habitat.

In 1901, there was a devastating epidemic of sleeping sickness in Uganda that killed some 250,000 people. A sleeping sickness commission was sent out to investigate, which included David Bruce, who had made his name discovering the cause of brucellosis (see Chapter 12). Bruce identified the rather beautiful trypanosome (pictured on the front cover of this book) that is the cause of both animal and human trypanosomiasis, and its transmission by the tsetse fly. With such an intractable vector, the only way to bring the epidemic to a close was to move the entire population away from the fly.

The species of fly found in East Africa, *Glossina morsitans*, ranges widely through the savannah, living in forest thickets and feeding on wild animals (especially bushbuck). Any humans brave enough to withstand its attack are likely to contract the more serious form of sleeping sickness caused by *Trypanosoma brucei rhodesiense*, which is found in this part of the continent. If not treated, this is invariably fatal, producing a progressively lethargic condition, much as its name suggests. As a result, large areas of East and southern Africa are unoccupied because of what is often called 'the curse of Africa'.

These unoccupied areas of Africa seem obvious places for settlement to the uninformed and are particularly tempting when you have a refugee problem on your hands. Such was the case in Tanzania with one of the many influxes of refugees from Rwanda/Burundi that has troubled these countries ever since they became independent.

In this particular instance, the first few cases of sleeping sickness appeared at the nearest hospital, all coming from Mishamo, the refugee settlement. When I visited Mishamo, I could see how well it had been set up, with a cleared area for all the buildings and good health facilities, but you did not need to be there long before you saw the odd tsetse fly powering its way through this new township. These flies, though, were just a few that had come out of the surrounding forest. In contrast, the journey to get to Mishamo was like driving through a war zone, with dive-bombers continually attacking your car, and if the tsetses managed to gain entrance, they inflicted their powerful bites on you when you were least expecting it. This was the area in which you were most likely to get infected due to the sheer number of bites, so it was mainly the hunter and honey collector, male occupations, that should have been the victims. However, something strange was happening, as most of the cases were in women and children, much more the pattern found in West Africa, where the tsetse flies through tunnels of forest along the course of rivers, biting anyone, particularly women that come to collect water. Normally, species of tsetse flies keep to their distinctive habitat, with those in West Africa quite different from those in the East, as in Tanzania, but here it seemed that a fly had crossed the ecological divide. So we conducted classic control measures as if the fly concerned was a West African species, clearing sections of forest along the course of rivers, especially around watering places, to break up the tunnel through which the flies travelled, and were gratified in bringing the epidemic to an end.

Plague and the Flea

Another disease transmitted by a vector that had considerable importance in history was that of plague. We tend to think of the Black Death and the epidemics of plague before it (see Chapter 5), as something that happened in the past, but all the components of a plague epidemic are present at this time. Plague exists in a focus in which the causative bacillus *Yersinia pestis*, its reservoir rodent and its vector flea are all present. Infection is maintained in a comparatively resistant colony of animals that do not seem to suffer unduly from disease. Their resident fleas transmit the organism from animal to animal, and as long as it is maintained in this resistant colony of animals, an epidemic of plague will not break out. These foci (Fig. 4.4) are found in various parts of the world and have persisted for considerable periods of time.

Up until quite recently, the bacillus responsible for causing plague was called *Pasteurella pestis* in honour of Louis Pasteur, but as Pasteur was never involved in investigating this particular disease, the organism has now more justifiably been called after Alexandre Yersin (1863–1943) the Swiss/French doctor who discovered the organism at the same time as Kitasato Shibasaburo during an epidemic in Hong Kong in 1894. (Debate continues as to who discovered it first, with proponents for and against in the home countries, but the majority side with Yersin.)

If it had not been for this discovery, Yersin would now have been remembered for his exploration of the Dong Nai River and Lang Bian Plateau, in what is now the central part of Vietnam, while he was serving as a ship's doctor on several vessels operating along the coast. He recommended that the future town of Da Lat be founded there, and the year after discovering the plague bacillus, set up a laboratory in Nha Trang that was to subsequently become the Pasteur Institute for the region. He prepared sera against plague, and also investigated cholera, smallpox and tetanus. Yersin is still honoured in Nha Trang, originally a town of the Cham empire, where his house is preserved as a museum. It contains a series of instruments he used to try to forecast approaching typhoons, so as to give the people time to take shelter. A remarkable man of many interests, he introduced the rubber tree (*Hevea brasiliensis*) and the quinine tree (*Cinchona ledgeriana*) to what was then French Indochina.

The foci of plague remain undisturbed in their own microhabitat, but if a human should wander into a focus and be accidentally bitten by a flea, such as from handling an animal that they have hunted or trapped, then they are liable to catch sylvatic plague, which occurs in rural wildlife. This presents as a swelling (a bubo, hence bubonic plague) of the regional lymph nodes draining the bite site and fever. If diagnosed early and treated, then the person will fully recover and no further cases develop. Isolated cases of sylvatic plague occur quite regularly in the USA, Mongolia and southern Russia.

A seasonal pattern of plague occurs in northern Tanzania in the otherwise lovely Usambara Mountains, centred on the favoured colonial retreat of Lushoto. This is an area where sugarcane is grown, which attracts the multimammate rat (*Mastomys natalensis*), which here is a reservoir of plague rather than of Lassa fever, as in West Africa. The rat feeds on the

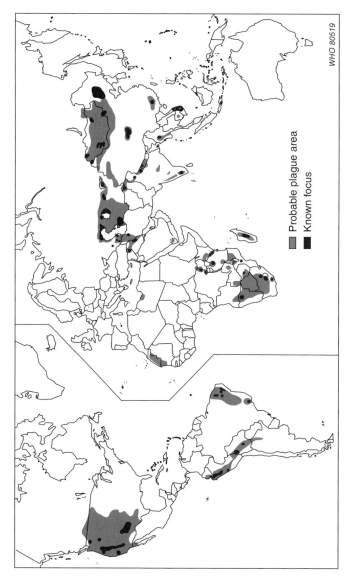

Fig. 4.4. Known and probable foci of plague. (Reproduced by permission of the World Health Organization, Geneva, Switzerland.)

stubble of the sugarcane after it has been harvested, but when this is burnt off in preparation for the next harvest, the hungry rats enter people's houses looking for food, which brings them into contact with the domestic rat, which is then fed upon by the plague-carrying fleas.

Often, the first sign of a plague outbreak is finding dead rats. This means that the fleas have now left the dead rats and are looking for another food source; the easiest option is for them to hop on to people, who then become the next victims. The obvious control strategy would seem to be to kill the rats, but in this dangerous situation, you are only encouraging the hungry fleas to move across and bite humans, who are very much their second choice as far as a source of food is concerned. So the fleas must be killed before the rats. This is done by blowing insecticide powder into burrows and clothing, as well as encouraging cleanliness and washing clothes with boiling water (or placing them overnight in a deep-freeze). These simple methods alone can be sufficient to bring an epidemic to a halt and it is tragic to think that, with this knowledge, the major epidemics that decimated the populations of Europe and Asia (see Chapter 5), could have been controlled.

Such is the complexity of plague that during an epidemic it is the rat flea, *Xenopsylla cheopis*, not the wild rodent flea, that is responsible for transmission. When it takes a blood meal, the plague bacilli multiply to such an extent in the crop of the flea that the feeding apparatus becomes blocked. When this so-called 'blocked flea' leaves a dead rat, it hops on to the nearest human, where it attempts to feed, but in the process injects plague bacilli into the unfortunate person. Frustrated from its attempt to acquire a blood meal, it moves on to another person, infecting them as well, and then continues in its attempts to feed off other people until it dies of hunger. The 'blocked flea' is therefore the main transmitter in the initial phases of an epidemic, and like the vector in filariasis, it is killed by the parasite it transmits.

Typhus and Its Vectors

Another disease similar to plague in not initially being an infection of humans is scrub typhus. Like wild rodent plague, scrub typhus is found in well-defined areas called mite islands, where the rodent, mite and infecting organism, *Rickettsia* or *Orientia*, live in a balance, with the rodent not appearing to show any undue illness from the infection. (The types of typhus and transmission cycles are illustrated in Fig. 4.5.)

The mite, which normally lives on a rodent, climbs on to grass and vegetation ready to cling to any passing animal, and if a human should be one of these, and the mite is infective, then they are liable to contract scrub typhus. This type of typhus (also known as tsutsugamushi fever) is often just a mild illness, and in rural areas where there are mite islands close to

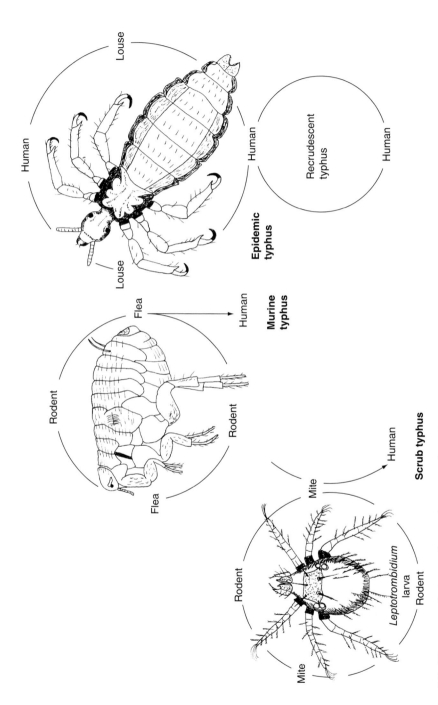

Fig. 4.5. The transmission cycles and vectors of scrub, murine and epidemic typhus. (From Webber, 2012, *Communicable Diseases: A Global Perspective*, 4th Edn.)

areas of habitation, people become used to developing a flu-like illness when they first move there.

Another form of typhus, called murine typhus, is associated more with towns, and its vector, the flea, is often the same flea as that responsible for most infections with plague, X. cheopis. (Much of the complex family of fleas was worked out and named by Lionel, 2nd Baron Rothschild, a member of the famous European banking dynasty, and founder of the Natural History Museum in London.) Murine typhus differs from scrub typhus in that it is the mammal that is the reservoir of infection, the flea just acting as the transmitter, but not by its bite. The causative organism, *Rickettsia typhi*, is found in the faeces of the flea, and it is the close association of humans with domestic rats, which have dried infected flea faeces in their fur, that causes transmission. An aerosol of organisms is sent into the air when the rat is disturbed, which is then inhaled, swallowed or absorbed through the conjunctiva.

In epidemic typhus, although the infecting organism is a *Rickettsia* (named after Howard Ricketts (1871–1910) the American pathologist who discovered the organism and tragically died of typhus while investigating an epidemic in Mexico City), there is no rodent involved in the cycle of transmission, only the human louse, *Pediculus humanus*. The *Rickettsia* is found in the faeces of the louse, and it is when the faeces are scratched into a bite wound, rubbed into the eye or accidentally swallowed, that infection takes place. Similarly, dried louse faeces form an aerosol when infested clothing is shaken, so organisms can be inhaled or swallowed by a person who does not have any lice on them.

Lice thrive in conditions of deprivation and poverty, where clothing is worn without being changed and people live in close proximity to each other, and they cannot travel far or survive for long without a blood meal. So it is the crowding together of people that allows the lice to crawl across and attach themselves to a new host. Such conditions as war, famine, prisons or refugee settlements provide the stage for an outbreak of typhus. A similar situation occurs in the highland areas of tropical countries – Burundi, Rwanda and Ethiopia in Africa, and Bolivia, Guatemala and Peru in the Americas. In 1997, there were 24,000 cases of epidemic typhus in Burundi.

Epidemic typhus is simply controlled by getting rid of body lice (not crab or pubic lice) by the use of insecticides applied to clothing and by encouraging people to wash. Placing clothes in a deep-freeze similarly kills off any lice or eggs in the clothing and it may well be that the ironing of clothes was first used historically as a means of killing lice, before its embellishment value was realized.

Typhus was first recorded in Spain in 1489, but it also added to the confusion of battle in the siege of Naples in 1528. It probably came to Spain with the Moorish invasion of the country, thus confirming its African origin, the part of the world where it is still predominantly found. This is further indicated by the African origin of the body louse, coinciding with early humans, as mentioned in Chapter 2.

Ticks

The other vector, more often associated with animals than viewed as a human problem, is the tick. We are used to finding the odd tick on our dogs and cats, and think they are just a nuisance, but the publicity around Lyme disease has brought the role of the tick, as the transmitter of diseases, more to our attention.

Lyme disease was so called because of cases of an encephalitic disease first described from Lyme, in Connecticut, USA. Infection is by a species of *Borellia*, and at least three different species are involved, hence the disease is also called borelliosis, especially in non-English speaking countries. It often starts with fever, headache and fatigue, and if untreated can go on to produce the more serious disease that involves the central nervous system. The herald sign is an expanding circular rash called erythema migrans, which appears at the bite site about a week after the tick has fallen off, and gradually increases in size, often with a clear area that makes it look like a target.

It is the very small nymphal stage of hard ticks of the genus *Ixodes* that are the main transmitter of disease, not the large adult tick that is more easily noticed. So after walking through country with tall grass or other vegetation from which the young tick can launch itself on to any passing animal, a search should be made for what looks like small black dots. There are many special devices invented for removing ticks, but as it is mainly the nymph that is important, these are quite unnecessary. An ordinary pair of tweezers, pulling the tick off as close to the skin as possible, and trying not to squeeze the body contents, is quite satisfactory. Ticks will remain attached for up to 36 hours and only about 1% of bites result in disease. Although it is mainly the deer tick in North America that transmits the infection, it is predominantly the sheep tick in Europe.

Despite the comparatively recent (1975) awareness of Lyme disease, it is a much older infection. Otzi the iceman was found to have a DNA sequence of *Borellia burgdorferi* that he must have acquired 5300 years ago when he was living in Alpine Europe. The first description of the illness was given by Rev. John Walker in 1764 from the island of Jura, off the West Coast of Scotland, from which people migrated between 1717 and the 19th century. The migration was due to the Scottish Clearance, with those from Jura predominantly going to the North Carolina region of the USA. The organism found a ready host in the ticks of North America, though it was originally a Euro/Asian disease.

The tick is also important in the transmission of some arboviral diseases (see Table 4.1.) as well as in tick-borne encephalitis (TBE), a disease that is increasingly occurring in the northern parts of Europe and Asia. The tick vector has recently extended its range into areas where it has not previously been found, in Germany, Scandinavia and Switzerland, as a consequence of climate change (see Chapter 17).

Vectors and Disease Selection

In this chapter, filariasis was described in perhaps more detail than would seem appropriate, but this was because it illustrates the conflict between natural selection and disease selection, but in a non-human situation. Natural selection favours the healthy female *Anopheles* mosquito to take blood meals on humans, to allow its eggs to develop, and so to continue the species. However, if it should take its blood meal from a filarial infected human, then it will be damaged by the parasite and be less fit. So the greater the number of humans infected with filariasis, the fewer healthy mosquitoes there will be to transmit other infections, including malaria. Disease selection therefore operates against the mosquito, but protects the uninfected human in which both malaria and filariasis are present at the same time in the population.

The Great Plagues

5

The Black Death

The first recorded case of germ warfare (bioterrorism) occurred in the Crimea in 1347 when the Mongols laid siege to the port of Caffa, now known as Feodosiya, at that time a Genovese stronghold. Unable to dislodge the defenders by ordinary means they catapulted into the fortress the dead bodies of victims of bubonic plague after the disease had broken out in their camp. The fleeing Genovese brought the disease to Messina in Sicily, where the plague broke out to start one of the greatest pandemics of all time, later called the Black Death.

The first cases of plague were the classical bubonic disease, as described in the previous chapter, in which the flea transmits the infection from one person to another. But in a few cases the infection attacked the respiratory system and the far more deadly form of pneumonic plague developed. This form of plague then became a respiratory infection, transferred directly from one person to another, which led to rapid spread and a high death rate.

By 1348, most of Europe was affected, and the plague crossed the English Channel to reach London later in that year to kill almost half of its 60,000 inhabitants. It spread throughout the whole country and reached Scotland by 1350. However, the effects of the disease were not homogenous, being worse in the towns and cities, where the proximity of large numbers of people favoured transmission, and relatively uncommon in rural areas.

The plague continued until 1353, spreading throughout Europe, North Africa and Asia as far as the Caspian Sea, killing nearly half the population and rewriting the demographic profile of its inhabitants. This was the largest decrease in population at any one time, far greater than any war or mass killing, and it cut right through every segment of the populace – both the old and the young, male and female, there was no particular pattern as to whom it attacked.

Those who had recovered and developed resistance, or had been able to escape to the country and isolated places to which infection never reached, were left to start the population again. As with so much of illness, it was the combination of poverty and overcrowding that permitted the greatest spread of the plague, so this was the major sector of the population devastated.

In the end, the epidemic died out because there were no longer sufficient susceptible people for infection to continue, but once the population had recovered, the scene was set for renewed epidemics in Europe over the next 300 years. Certainly there were domestic rats and fleas to restart transmission, but there were no established foci of plague (as previously described in Chapter 4; see Fig. 4.4.), so it is probable that temporary foci involving rodents, their fleas and the bacilli were established.

In many ways, the Black Death was the end of the period known as the Middle Ages. This was not so much a calendar period but the feudal system that had been the structure of society. Large estates were passed on by hereditary rites, and the majority of the population worked for their lords and masters, giving a tithe of the food produced and becoming soldiers in times of war. With the devastation of the population, there was not the same labour force to maintain the estates, and the indiscriminate plague had also cut down the ruling elite just as easily. So the plague brought about a complete change from the feudal system, in which a money economy developed both for the purchase of land and the employment of people to work on it. Those of ability, even from a humble background, had the opportunity to rise to positions of power – the peasant could become the country gent. Other means of making money – business and the service industry – developed, heralding the birth of the modern age.

It was not just in Europe that plague changed the order of rule, but also in the other great civilization of the world, China. The magnificent Ming Dynasty was brought to an untimely end by plague in 1644. Faced with attacks from barbarian nations on all sides, its armies were reduced so catastrophically by plague that it could not mount an adequate defence. The physician responsible for treating the troops was the first person to realize that pneumonic plague was spread as a respiratory infection, and he imposed quarantine regulations to try to isolate these cases. Sadly, his successes were not sufficient to turn the tide of history.

It was the epidemic of plague in China that led to the last great European epidemic, ironically known as the Renaissance plague, in 1665–1666. In England, it particularly devastated London, where 15% of the population, some 68,595 people, were said to have died. This was mainly due to the chaotic way in which the situation was handled, with corpses being buried in mass graves or wherever a place could be found.

The Great Fire of London brought the epidemic to an end as it burnt its way through the many thatched roofs that were ideal breeding places for rats. Regulations dictated that all roofs on the new houses to be built should be of slate to reduce the fire risk but, unknowingly, this was probably one of the most important public health interventions ever implemented in the capital.

In 1665, Isaac Newton, after receiving his degree from Trinity College, Cambridge, returned home to escape the plague. Contemplating what he had learnt and with little to do, it was reputed that it was while he was relaxing in his garden that he had his revolutionary inspiration about gravity. As to whether it was due to 'the falling apple' is speculation, but more certain is the fact that it was the plague, which had driven him to the countryside, that was responsible for the idea that was to change the world.

As a postscript, it may be noted that the first recorded epidemic of plague, the Justinian plague, was in Constantinople in AD 542, and this was to change the course of history just as profoundly as the Black Death did centuries later. The Emperor Justinian had succeeded in reconquering Italy, Spain and much of North Africa to reaffirm the Roman Empire, but the plague so decimated the population, killing perhaps 100 million, that it left a power vacuum to be filled by the growing armies of Islam. So it was disease rather than the doctrine of a new religion that changed the fate of this part of the world.

Smallpox

It would seem almost certain that smallpox came out of Africa with our earliest ancestors, as it has been found on Egyptian mummies and was recorded in their literature. In addition, there is a group of animal pox diseases, including monkeypox, which suggests that the human disease may have developed from it. Smallpox, which is caused by an *Orthopoxvirus*, is one of the most contagious diseases ever known; unlike plague, you could not run away to your country retreat to escape. It spared no one in its progress through the population, bringing to an end the lives of the great and wealthy as much as those of the poorer classes.

Smallpox starts with a fever and rash of quite sudden onset, leaving the victim prostrated. The rash was the characteristic feature of the disease, but had to be differentiated from that of chickenpox, with which it might initially be confused. As medical students, we were taught that the 'C' of chickenpox reminded us of the characteristic 'central' distribution of the rash. Also, the skin lesions of chickenpox, which become progressively papules, vesicles and pustules, are found in different stages, rather than all going through the same stage at the same time, as is seen in smallpox.

In contrast, the smallpox sufferer was characteristically very ill and had a rash predominantly on the extremities of the face, limbs and hands (with pox lesions on the palms and soles of the feet being particularly diagnostic), all the lesions passed through the same stage at the same time, and in the vesicle stage they were deep seated, flat topped and depressed in the middle. The fever intensified as the rash progressed to the pustular stage, which was the very worst time for the person. They felt terrible, their skin was an oozing mass, they could not eat or drink because of spots inside their mouths and they just wanted to die, which is what happened to large numbers of them. If they recovered from this severe stage, the sores left deep marks, especially on the sides of the face, so that the sufferer was marked for life. While this meant that they were immune to repeat infection, it was a disfigurement that spoilt the chance of marriage for many a good-looking girl.

For smallpox to develop into an epidemic, a sufficient number of people is required for the virus (*Variola major*) to pass easily from one person to another. The first epidemics were recorded in the early civilizations of Egypt, Mesopotamia and the Indus Valley. This has given rise to the alternative theory of the virus having been transferred to humans from the pox diseases of camels and gerbils, to which *V. major* is more closely related than it is to the monkeypox virus. However, these first epidemics might also have occurred because of the concentrated nature of these populations, and their ability to record the outbreaks in their histories, for it is not until the next great civilization, that of the Greeks, that smallpox appears again. The description of the plague of Athens in 430 BC is more characteristic of smallpox than of bubonic plague, and from Athens it spread into the rest of Europe, decimating any concentrations of population.

In Europe in the Middle Ages, it was the church that ran the early hospitals and treated the sick, so it is in their records that we find the first descriptions of smallpox, such as that by Bishop Gregory of an epidemic in AD 580 that raged through Italy and southern France:

> A person, after being seized with a violent fever, was covered all over with vesicles and small pustules which were white, hard, unyielding and very painful. If the patient survived to their maturation, they broke and began to discharge, when the pain was greatly increased by the adhesion of the clothes of the body…nor any part of the body remained exempt…[even the] eyes were wholly closed up.

Any part of the skin lesions, the vesicle fluid, the pus or the scabs contained the smallpox virus, so infection could be transferred from these. This was reasonably obvious to a relative or attendant looking after the sick person, but most infections probably resulted from coughing, when the virus was spread through the air to the unsuspecting contact. It then only needed a concentration of people for the virus to spread from one person to another, and in so doing relentlessly work its way through the population.

Elizabeth I had only been queen for 4 years when she was laid low by smallpox. She had famously declared herself to be the 'Virgin Queen', who would concentrate all of her abilities on being a great ruler rather than on concerns of partnership, marriage and producing children. As such, she had no direct descendant and it would most likely have been her Catholic cousin, Mary Queen of Scots, who would have taken her place, should she have died. Memories of Elizabeth's older sister Mary were still fresh in people's minds – memories of the terrible tortures and sufferings that she inflicted on the burgeoning Protestant population, as she sought to turn the country back to Catholicism. Nobody wanted this again, so the country went into retreat, prayers were offered for the Queen's recovery and there was no other subject so discussed as the monarch's malady when, to everybody's relief, she recovered. Perhaps, though, the scars were always with her, as one of the theories put forward for her heavy use of make-up, applied to such an extent that it was caked white on her face, was to hide the pox marks that lay beneath.

Although the Stuarts did succeed Elizabeth, with Mary's son James, as a dynasty, they were not so fortunate in escaping from the dangers of the pox. James's son Charles I lost his head to the axe but it was the smallpox that killed a brother and sister of his grandson, Charles II. This left the order of succession to Charles's unpopular Catholic brother, James II, who was forced to abdicate in favour of his daughter, Mary, when the wrath of the people so opposed his attempts to change the religion of the land back to Catholicism. Mary was married to the great Protestant protector of Europe, William of Orange, who became joint monarch of England with his wife. Sadly, Mary died of smallpox before she produced an heir, so her sister Anne became queen after William. She, however, was to be the last of the Stuart monarchs because her son died from smallpox while he was still a boy. The Scottish dynasty was replaced by the Hanoverians, who traced their legitimacy through Sophia of Palatinate, a granddaughter of James I, but by then it was purely a matter of the right to succeed rather than to be part of the royal house that had replaced the Tudors.

Smallpox can justly claim to have changed the course of British history, as it did of the Austrian, French, Russian, Spanish and Swedish royal families as well, by killing off various kings, queens and emperors. It was possibly also the cause of death of one of the Egyptian pharaohs, Ramses V, as when his mummy was critically examined by electron microscopy, virus particles similar to those of smallpox were discovered. Furthermore, smallpox was to cross the Atlantic and change the history of South and Central America, as will be covered in Chapter 8.

Perhaps the Indians should be given the credit for the practice of inoculation against smallpox, although it is best known from Turkey. Needles dipped in pus from a smallpox pustule were used to puncture the skin, generally on the upper arm of children. Some 8 days later, the children felt unwell, with the appearance of a few pocks, but they did not get the major illness or scarring, and were protected for the rest of their lives.

Lady Mary Montague, wife of the British ambassador to the Ottoman Empire, heard about the practice when she travelled to Constantinople (now Istanbul) in 1716. Having suffered from smallpox herself, she had her son inoculated without any ill effect, so when the family returned to England in 1721, at the same time as a smallpox epidemic was raging, she had her daughter inoculated as well. The protection of her children against smallpox was witnessed by several eminent physicians, but there was still concern that the procedure was not without its dangers. It had been tried on only a few people, so there was always the risk of serious disease developing in a minority, in addition to the live virus spreading and initiating new epidemics. Despite these risks inoculation became a common practice, as death from smallpox was in the region of 20%, whereas that from inoculation just over 1%. Today this would be an unacceptable risk for the well child, so it was fortunate that an English country physician made one of the most important observations in medical history.

Edward Jenner (1749–1823) lived in Berkeley, Gloucestershire and, like many of the doctors of his day, was as interested in natural history as he was in the practice of medicine. He was an astute observer, inspired by his apprenticeship to the famous surgeon and anatomist John Hunter. It was Hunter's dictum 'Why think, why not try the experiment?' that was to prove the most important advice he ever received.

Jenner noticed that milkmaids did not develop smallpox as they commonly contracted cowpox, a mild infection. He came to realize that not only did cowpox protect against smallpox, but it could be used as a deliberate way of protecting people from the more serious infection. So in 1796, Jenner took fluid from the blisters of fresh cowpox lesions of a young dairymaid, Sarah Nelmes, and inoculated the 8-year-old James Phipps. The boy developed a low-grade fever and minor lesion from which he soon recovered. There was a smallpox outbreak almost 2 months later, so Jenner took some smallpox pus and inoculated James, who remained completely well. Jenner sent a paper to the Royal Society describing the experiment, but it was rejected; so after several more vaccination experiments he privately published *An Inquiry into the Causes and Effects of the Variolae Vaccinae, a Disease Known by the Name of Cow Pox*.

With such a title, it is perhaps not surprising that this groundbreaking work was not immediately hailed as a major breakthrough, but some doctors were quick to grasp the potential and, as so often happens, tried to take the credit for themselves. Gradually, the practice of vaccination, as it came to be called (after the *V. vaccinae* of cowpox), spread to the rest of Europe and to America. There was, though, the problem of obtaining fresh fluid from cowpox lesions, as Jenner had recommended that vaccine material be obtained from the pox lesions of a vaccinated child, thereby allowing a continuous supply. However, this was not necessarily available to the casual vaccinator, so some of the vaccinations that were done were not reliable. It was not until methods of growing the vaccine were developed that safe vaccination could be ensured. Smallpox rapidly declined in countries that had instituted vaccination, but then reappeared later as a disease of adults, so it was realized that one dose of vaccine did not give lifelong protection, but had to be repeated.

Jenner himself had suggested that smallpox could finally be annihilated, so just less than 200 years after his momentous experiment, the World Health Organization (WHO) launched the Worldwide Smallpox Eradication Campaign in 1966. This stressed universal vaccination to a level of over 80%, the isolation of cases and the tracing of all contacts of a case. Considering there were wars continuing in several countries, making vaccination coverage difficult, as well as religious objections and many other problems, it is a considerable triumph that eradication was finally certified on 9 October 1979, some 2 years after the last case of naturally acquired disease was found.

Changing History

The great plagues almost threatened our species. If it had not been for the variety of individuals (due to the original pressure from disease resulting in the production of two sexes, as discussed in Chapter 1), with a few people able to survive, some communities, if not larger groupings of people, might not have been able to recover. Although humans survived, disease changed history in a radical way: whole nation states disappeared and the order of life was never to be the same again.

Missionaries of Death

6

Samoa

John Williams, the great missionary from the London Missionary Society (LMS), had achieved remarkable success in converting most of the Polynesian people to Christianity. Within just a few years, he had seen the transformation of these distant Pacific Islanders from war-mongering cannibals to passive Christians. Now he was to turn his attention to the much bigger challenge of the Melanesian (meaning 'black') Islands. He felt sure he was going to succeed: against all odds he had done so in Samoa (Fig. 6.1), he had God on his side, soon he would be able to claim even greater numbers of converts to the religion he so believed in.

He had chosen to launch his crusade on the island of Tanna, part of what was then called the New Hebrides, so named by Captain Cook, who was probably thinking of places nearer home. Williams left a couple of his missionaries to learn the language and then proceeded to Erromanga (now Erromango) to do the same. However, when he went ashore he was immediately clubbed to death, so it is not on the coral islands of Polynesia that the great missionary is buried, but on Erromanga that his grave is to be found. It is likely that he was thought to be a sandalwooder, one of the unscrupulous exploiters of the precious sandalwood, so landing unarmed made him easy prey.

Among the Melanesian people land is owned by the community, but every part of it – every hill, every rock, even every tree – has significance. Trees in particular serve as markers, often believed to be inhabited by spirits, so to fell a tree is a major evil. Armed loggers came from Australia and essentially stole the sandalwood trees, probably killing any of the people who tried to stop them, so any white-skinned person was immediately suspected of being a logger.

The shock of John Williams's death reverberated around the Pacific and the people of Erromanga received a very bad reputation but, in reality, they might have done themselves a considerable service. On John

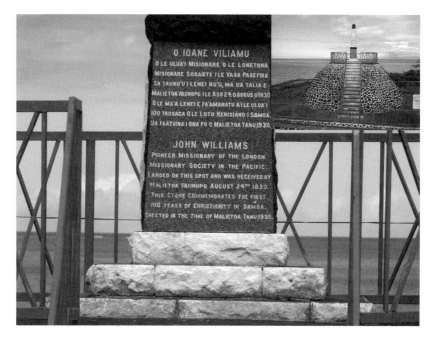

Fig. 6.1. The John Williams memorial at Sapapalii, on the island of Savai'i, Samoa. It commemorates his first landing to introduce Christianity, but there is no mention of the influenza epidemic that was unleashed and killed large swathes of the population.

Williams's ship when he first landed in Samoa was a more deadly passenger, influenza, which spread through the Pacific Islands like wildfire. The people had never met the virus before and it devastated the population as a killer disease. Indeed, it probably helped the conversion process, as the missionary could forgive the dying person their sins and tell them they would go to heaven – both purgatory and its redeemer coming at the same time.

John Williams's ship was called the *Messenger of Peace*, but should perhaps have been called the *Messenger of Death*, such was the havoc that it wrought. When it came to Erromanga, the people did not let the same thing happen again. John Williams might have met his end, but the people of Erromanga inadvertently prevented many of their people from going the same way.

Fiji

It was not influenza but measles that came to Fiji. Measles is normally a childhood disease, but because the people had not been in contact with it before, all ages were affected at the same time. This was particularly serious because the adults were too ill to look after their children, so many died unnecessarily, when with good nursing and careful feeding they may have survived.

The measles epidemic of 1875 killed a quarter of the population of Fiji. Whole families and every level of society was affected, resulting in a high death rate. In fact, the population was so depleted that it never properly recovered.

One immediate effect of this was the so-called Kai Colo Wars (1875–1876), which resulted from the dissatisfaction of the interior people of Viti Levu (the main island) with the signing of the Deed of Cession to Great Britain of 1874, as they had not been consulted. The measles epidemic was viewed by the Kai Colo people (of the interior) as witchcraft, in collusion with their traditional enemies, the coastal people, to destroy them. Hostilities ensued and it took until Chief Kunati's impregnable Hill Fort near Sigatoka was stormed, and he was killed, that peace finally came in 1876.

The economy of Fiji is mainly from sugar and in colonial times indentured labour was brought from India to cut the sugarcane. This was partly due to the loss of labour that had resulted from the epidemic, but also because the indigenous Fijians were the landowners. While the Fijian population only slowly recovered from the epidemic, that of the expatriate Indians increased at a greater rate, with the result that they now outnumber the original inhabitants. Many of the Indians went into business, so not only did they become the majority population, but now much of the wealth belonged to them too. However, the land was still held by the traditional Fijian society and could not be bought, leading to friction between the two communities. This was further accentuated during elections that gave the majority (Fijian) Indian population the balance of power. Twice the military has taken over power to preserve the rights of the traditional Fijians, and this disparity continues to be a problem to the present day.

In Fiji, the disease of measles not only devastated the population, but changed the balance of power and altered the government of the country. Disease had certainly selected against the naturally selected inhabitants of these islands.

Nauru

The island of Nauru is the smallest nation in the world (except for the Vatican City which holds rather a special position as far as nation states go), and is in a strategic position between the islands of the South Pacific and those of the North Pacific. When phosphate was discovered, for a brief period between the 1960s and 1970s the people of Nauru became the richest per capita nation in the world. Such was their wealth that they invested in property in Australia and had their own airline, which provided a very useful service by flying between the islands of the North and South Pacific.

Nauru became a German territory in 1888, when not only did they receive their first administrators from Germany, but also their first missionaries, who set about converting them to Christianity. Fortunately, there seems to be no reason for blaming them for the introduction of diseases, as it was not until 1920 that influenza was introduced, as part of the worldwide pandemic. As in other Pacific Islands, the disease ripped through the population, giving an 18% mortality rate.

It is, however, not influenza that makes Nauru such a unique story as far as disease is concerned, but leprosy. This was an ancient disease in Europe and Asia, where the populations had gradually developed immunity, and so the disease ceased to be a problem by the early 20th century. In contrast, this was not the case in developing countries and in island populations that had kept themselves free of contact from the rest of the world. How leprosy was introduced to Nauru is not known, but between 1921 and 1925 an epidemic of the disease raged that affected 30% of the population.

Leprosy is normally a chronic disease, with a spectrum of symptom complexes extending from lepromatous leprosy at one extreme to tuberculoid leprosy at the other (see Chapter 1). This is the pattern found in most countries, even those that have only become infected in comparatively recent times, but it is always found in endemic form. To have an epidemic in such a chronic infection is very unusual, and Nauru is one of the few places that such an epidemic has ever been recorded. All ages were susceptible to the disease, with most people fortunately developing the tuberculoid type of the disease, so that after it had passed through the population it gradually died out. There is no sign of it now, but as a natural experiment in leprosy, Nauru is unique.

Interestingly this tiny country has another claim to fame in the world of disease, in having one of the highest rates of diabetes of any country. During their period of affluence – and this was a shared affluence, because Micronesian society distributes its wealth through family relationships, and nearly everybody was related – every person had a right to their share, and people just spent and spent. You would see supermarket trolleys absolutely laden with food, with the consequence that the rate of obesity was almost 100%. However, it was probably not the obesity alone, but a genetic adaptation that had stood them in good stead in the past, that now came back to give them trouble.

The Polynesian and Micronesian peoples are the greatest sailors the world has ever known. They set off, probably from what is now Indonesia into the North Pacific, and from the eastern Solomon Islands and Banks Islands into the South Pacific. The first journey that Columbus made was just a fraction of the distance that these people had travelled into the unknown, and this was many hundreds of years later. They sailed in ocean-going canoes, had an incredible knowledge of the sea and somehow reached distant islands many months later. The first island group they reached was Fiji, which they inhabited from about 1500 BC. From here groups of pioneers continued on to Samoa and Tonga, eventually to find every island in the vastness of the Pacific by AD 900.

To be able to achieve these incredible journeys, virtually on starvation rations and what they could harvest from the sea, the people adapted to keeping going on a marginal blood-sugar level. But once this was no longer necessary, and especially when the reverse happened and they had far more food than they required, their blood-sugar level went through the roof. These people mainly suffer from type 2 (or adult-onset) diabetes, which has a rising rate with age. A first survey conducted in 1975 found that 34.4% of the population had diabetes. Since this wake-up call, efforts have been made to reduce the incidence of diabetes by getting people to cut down on the amount of sugar and total food that they eat, as well as by campaigns to reduce smoking, so that by the time of the 2004 survey the overall incidence had decreased to 16.24%. However, the increase of the incidence rate with age continued, such that those in the 55–64 years age group had an overall rate of 45%, which was 52.8% in women of this age group and 37.4% in men. Diabetes continues to be the major health concern in this small Pacific nation.

Africa

The missionaries that went to Africa suffered the reverse fate of those in the Pacific; instead of being the ones that brought disease and its consequences, they were the ones that succumbed to it. To go to Africa, one was almost certain to contract malaria and, in areas of high transmission such as West Africa, the mortality rate was enormous. Some Europeans did obtain immunity by using judicious doses of quinine and wearing protective clothing, while others discovered less malarious areas, such as the highlands and drier parts of the country, to establish their mission stations. So to be a missionary was just as much about inadvertently killing off others as being killed yourself; it just depended on which part of the world you went to.

The Value of Immunity

Natural selection favoured a group of hardy seafarers to populate the distant islands of the Pacific. To survive for long periods at sea and successfully navigate to small land masses was a major asset to the people who inhabited the furthest extremities of the globe. But these assets were of no value though when challenged by introduced diseases, resulting in considerable mortality. Fortunately, the immune mechanisms that had saved their ancestors in the competition with disease were able to help them to survive this new challenge.

The Slave Trade in Parasites 7

Hookworm Disease

Between 1910 and 1914, the Rockefeller Foundation undertook a massive campaign to rid the southern states of the USA from hookworm disease. There was a reasonably effective treatment and by giving it to as much of the population as possible it was hoped to free the country from this debilitating disease.

The hookworm lives in the intestines where the adult worm invaginates a piece of mucosa from which it extracts blood and nutrients. Eggs are passed in the faeces and they hatch into larvae in the soil after 8–10 days to produce the infective form, which is able to pierce the skin of the foot in the generally unshod individual (Fig. 7.1). Once the larva has managed to penetrate the skin, it migrates to a blood or lymphatic vessel, where it is carried to the lungs, and breaking out through the alveolar wall, it passes up through the trachea and down the oesophagus, back into the intestines. Despite this extensive journey through the body, the hookworm causes no serious damage and it is only within the gut, where it develops into an adult, that it causes any pathological changes. A few worms are no problem, indeed might even confer benefit (see Chapter 14), but a heavy load can lead to anaemia, and in the young child be the determinant of survival into adult life. Some 60–120 worms will produce slight anaemia, whereas over 300 worms, coupled with malnutrition, could be sufficient to kill the child.

There are two species of hookworms that infect humans, *Ancylostoma duodenale* and *Necator americanus*, which are distinguished by the shape of their mouthparts (Fig. 7.1). The irony is that the common hookworm found in the southern USA and called *N. americanus*, as this was where it was first described, is most likely to have come from Africa, so perhaps should more rightly be called *N. africanus*. Carried in the early slaves who were transported across the Atlantic, the hookworm soon found the ideal conditions of temperature and soil type (sandy/loam) to spread among the resident population.

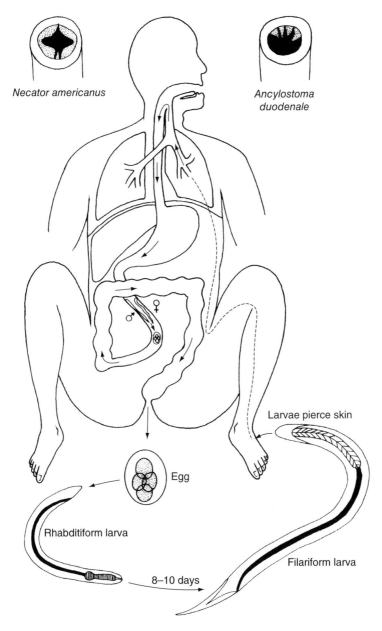

Fig. 7.1. The hookworm life cycle and its identification from the mouthparts. (From Webber, 2012, *Communicable Diseases: A Global Perspective*, 4th Edn.)

Getting people to wear shoes was probably the most effective way of interrupting transmission, but the heroic efforts of the Rockefeller Foundation would have helped considerably to reduce the worm load. Now, with the general acceptance of wearing shoes and using toilets, the infection has been controlled, but at the time the slaves certainly brought their revenge with them.

Schistosomiasis

The 16th to 19th centuries saw some of the largest movements in population due to the international slave trade. Much is known about the slave trade from the western part of Africa, but there was also an extensive trade from the east, which went to the countries of the Arabian Peninsula (Fig. 7.2).

The main need for slaves was as labourers in the sugar and cotton industries, so it was to the southern USA, the Caribbean and the north-eastern part of South America that the slaves were transported. These then were the parts of the world that offered possible environments for new diseases to take hold.

Schistosomiasis (also called bilharziasis after Bilharz who first found the parasite in Egypt in 1851) is a disease transmitted by a fluke, a large parasite, which depending on its species, is found in different parts of the body. The parasite found by Bilharz is now known as *Schistosoma haematobium* and lives in the bladder where, as its name suggests, it causes bleeding, which presents as blood in the urine. Another form of the parasite, *S. mansoni*, was named after Sir Patrick Manson (see Chapter 4). The third form is known as *S. japonicum* as it was first found in a patient in Japan, but it should probably have been called *S. sinensis*, as it has a longer history in China.

The tomb of the Marquess of Dai (Xin Zui) in Changsha was remarkably well preserved when it was accidentally discovered in 1972, allowing detailed study of her mummified remains, which were dated to 160 BC. She managed to live into her 50s despite suffering from tuberculosis, gall stones, arteriosclerosis and schistosomiasis. As Changsha is situated on a tributary of the Yangtze, it is likely that schistosomiasis was endemic throughout most of the great river's course.

S. mansoni and *S. japonicum* live in the intestinal tissues, but also migrate into the liver where they can cause liver fibrosis and serious liver damage. *S. haematobium* damages the bladder and ureters, but can also lead to the development of bladder cancer. All forms of the disease require a water snail intermediate host and it is this that determines where the infection will take hold. Eggs passed in the faeces from *S. mansoni* and *S. japonicum*, and in the urine from *S. haematobium* – the only multicelled parasite that transmits infection by the urine – develop into an active form (called a miracidium) which searches out a snail of a particular species. In the snail, the miracidia undergo changes to emerge as the infective forms, called a cercaria, which will penetrate through the skin of anybody that enters the water. From the skin, the cercariae go through developmental stages in the body to become adult males and females in the intestines and bladder, respectively.

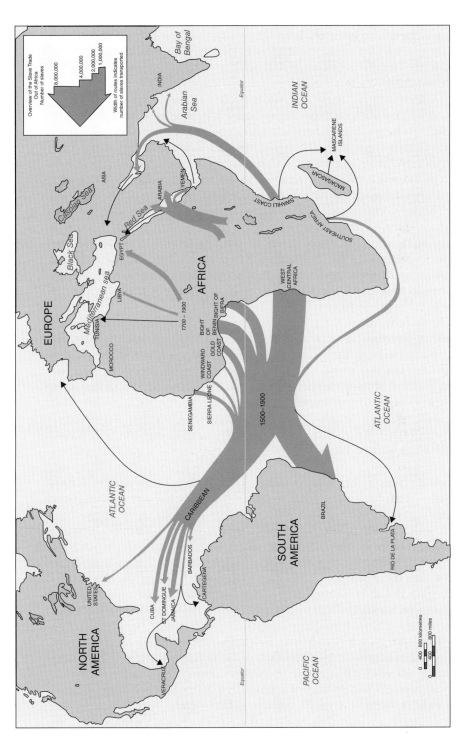

The complexity of the life cycle is considerable, with less than 50% of the eggs able to leave the bladder or intestines – it is the eggs trapped in the tissues that cause most of the damage. They must enter water, which needs to be between 10 and 30°C, and have sufficient light to induce hatching. The miracidia must find the right kind of snail within 8–12 hours, with only some 40% of snails becoming infected in still water at a distance of 5 m. Cercariae are stimulated to emerge from the snail by daylight, reaching a peak between 12.00 hours and mid-to-late afternoon, depending on the species. They then have 24 hours to find and penetrate a person, and have an increasing rate of mortality the longer it takes them, with 50% dying by 8 hours. Yet despite this, schistosomiasis is a common infection in much of the world, as seen in Fig. 7.3.

The snail intermediate hosts of the disease are species specific, with *S. haematobium* requiring members of the *Bulinus* snail genus, *S. mansoni* requiring *Biomphalaria* and *S. japonicum* the very hardy *Oncomelania*. When slaves were carried from West Africa across the Atlantic, they carried their *S. mansoni* with them and in many of the Caribbean Islands, the Guianas, Venezuela and Brazil, the parasites found *Biomphalaria* snails for the disease to take up residence (Fig. 7.3).

From East Africa, *S. mansoni* was carried to the Arabian Peninsula and *S. haematobium* to Yemen and Iraq. Because *S. haematobium* was first discovered in Egypt and there are ancient Egyptian mummies with evidence of the disease, it is possible that it spread to these countries in more ancient times, but its wide distribution would still suggest that the slave trade played a part in transferring it.

Filariasis in the New World

There are two types of filarial infection and both of these appear to have travelled with their slave hosts to set up residence in South America and the Caribbean. The first, lymphatic filariasis (see Chapter 4), predominantly a disease of Africa, has reached many parts of the world, but by its distribution in the Caribbean Islands, Hispaniola (Haiti and the Dominican Republic) and the Atlantic coast of South America indicates that it was disseminated to this part of the world during the slave trade. Indeed, in Brazil, it is found only in the north-east, around Recife, where much of the slave traffic was directed. The species that is responsible in this area is *Wucheria bancrofti*.

The other type of filarial infection is that produced by *Onchocerca volvulus*, which affects the skin and the eyes, eventually leading to blindness, giving it the alternative name of river blindness. The disease is particularly serious in West Africa but extends in a belt across the tropical centre of Africa as far as Malawi. *O. volvulus* is transmitted by small biting flies called *Simulium* which, despite their size, inflict a painful bite and have the

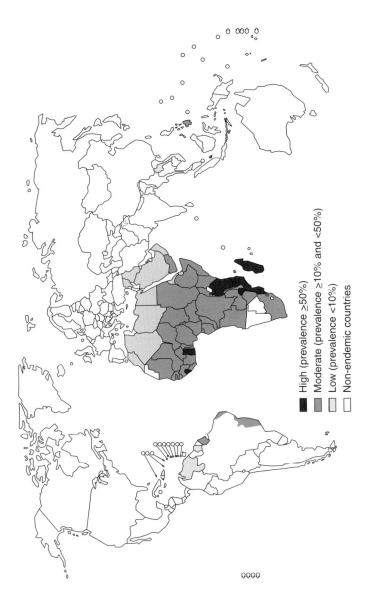

Fig. 7.3. Global distribution of schistosomiasis in 2009. (Reproduced by permission of the World Health Organization, Geneva, Switzerland.)

persistence of a mosquito or midge. These breed in fast-flowing streams, typical of mountainous areas, so it is only where the *Simulium* fly is found that foci of infection develop.

As parts of South and Central America and Yemen are the only places outside Africa where the disease occurs, it would seem likely that it arrived there from Africa via infected slaves. Yemen was also a destination for slaves from East Africa, and had the mountainous and fast-flowing streams that are required by the vector, so the occurrence of the disease here adds to the evidence that infection travelled with the slaves. In the Americas, although the distribution is not that of the main places that slaves were introduced, many of them ran away to live in the jungle, not too dissimilar to the African forests from which they had come. Pursued by the slave owners, they went deeper and deeper into the interior, where there was the opportunity for local *Simulium* flies to feed on them and become infected. Many of the South and Central American foci of this type of filariasis have now been eliminated, so one of the diseases introduced by slaves has been brought to an end.

The Jigger

The best recorded account of a disease transmitted by the slave trade is unusual in that it happened the other way round.

Fleas normally attach to the outside of the body, where they take their blood meal and cause irritable bites. However one species of flea, *Tunga penetrans*, actually burrows into the skin. After it has been fertilized, the female penetrates the skin, usually in the feet. The part of the foot where the flea penetrates swells as the eggs develop in the flea's body, to form what is called a jigger (or chigoe). These can be excruciatingly painful and are also a passage for bacterial infection to enter and produce an ulcer. Fortunately, they are easily removed with a pin, and some local people develop expertise in getting them out in a complete piece.

Jiggers were first described by the Spanish in 1525, although they were found predominantly in Portuguese-speaking Brazil. In terms of seriousness, they are little more than a nuisance, but as they are one of those infections – similar to the larvae of certain flies that bore their way into the body – they cause more anxiety and worry and attract greater attention than other problems, hence they were written about by the Spanish.

Having delivered its cargo of slaves, the British ship *Thomas Mitchell* returned from Rio de Janeiro to Angola in 1872 for a further shipment. A sailing ship must have sufficient ballast, so that when the wind hits its sails it does not capsize. This is especially necessary when the holds are empty of their cargo, so to compensate, ballast in the form of rocks or, in this particular case, sand had been loaded. Once the ship arrived in Angola, it discharged its ballast, which unfortunately carried eggs of *T. penetrans.*

The soil type in this part of Angola was perfect for its development and the barefoot African the ideal host.

From Angola, the flea travelled with the slave caravans deep into the interior of Africa and was soon being spread in the indigenous population. Zanzibar was the main slave market on the East African coast, and it took only 25 years after its introduction into Angola for the jigger to cross Africa and infect slaves from this part of the continent. It is now endemic in Africa, where it produces much misery, especially in children and the poor.

Other Movements of Slaves

The African slave trade was not the first time that people had been enslaved in such large numbers. Slavery was practised by the Romans, the Mongols and all of the Islamic dynasties.

The people that are now known as Slavs obtained their name from being taken as slaves – Slav is a word derived from the Greek meaning slave. Huge numbers were used in the mines by the Romans and others absorbed into the army. This caused a major change in the population of Europe.

The Mongols created the largest land empire in the history of the world by defeating and enslaving many of the people in the vast area they conquered. Countless were killed or moved to other parts of the empire, causing major ethnic and demographic changes in the population of Asia.

Slavery was part of the way of life of the Abbasid caliphate of Baghdad, which unwittingly brought to power a group of people who were formerly slaves. As a group, they were known as *mamluk*, which interprets as 'owned'. These slaves were taken from the nomadic Turkic people of Central Asia, who because of their military qualities were used as bodyguards and military personnel throughout the caliphate. However, they later overthrew their rulers to conquer much of the eastern Mediterranean, extending into Syria by AD 877. The first Mameluke dynasty lasted until AD 905, but they again rose to power in 1250 to famously defeat the Mongols in 1260.

We do not know the effects of disease within these slave movements, but it is likely that there were transfers of infectious conditions similar to those that had happened from Africa. There were certainly huge demographic changes and an intermingling of different genes, thereby increasing genetic diversity and the advantages that this brought in combating disease.

Eden's Garden of South America

8

The Peopling of America

The biggest controversy in archaeology is over the time when humans first entered the Americas. Established work in North America decided this was about 15,000–17,000 years ago, based on the Clovis culture, for which there are dated artefacts up to 13,000 BP (years before present). Furthermore, 80% of the present North American populations have genetic links to the Clovis people. However, sites in Chile at Cueva Fell and Monte Verde suggest that people migrated into South America at a much earlier date. There have been remarkable findings at Pedra Furada (now called the Serra da Capivara National Park), where remains have been dated to 17,000–32,000 BP. Not only do these dates considerably antedate those of the Clovis culture, but Serra da Capivara is in Brazil, inland from Recife, on the east side of South America, thus suggesting that ancient peoples travelled into what is now the Amazon, as well as following down the Pacific coast, as had always been presumed.

The Monte Verde site in Chile is dated to 14,000 to 14,600 years ago, so for humans to have reached this far south would indicate that they entered America between 16,000 and 20,000 years ago, probably along the Pacific coast of North America. Tantalizing evidence from the Queen Charlotte Islands in British Columbia lends support to this route, although much evidence would have been destroyed by the changes in sea level produced by the last Ice Age. Interestingly, nine varieties of seaweed were found during the Monte Verde excavations, suggesting that they were used as local medicines, as now practised by the present-day Mapuche Indians. Seaweed is a source of iodine and prevents the development of goitre, and these resourceful ancestors have also produced the first evidence of eating wild potatoes (*Solanum maglia*).

When early man entered South America, it was like entering a new world. Although humans had become cold adapted – crossing the ice bridge between Siberia and Alaska – they now entered a warmer land, abundant with animals and other food sources, a veritable Garden of Eden. Even the Amazon was not the dense jungle that it is today; with the climate then it was more like the savannah of East Africa or the present fringing forest around Boa Vista in the northern part of Brazil. What was more, it was virtually disease free, as there had been no chance for parasites to adapt to the new invaders, and with a change in the climate, the diseases of colder regions (particularly chest infections) were now less of a problem to them.

Introduction of Old World Diseases

This happy state of affairs was allowed to continue up until the arrival of Europeans in the 15th century, as populations such as the Incas and several of the great civilizations that preceded them had more than enough people living closely together for any of the well-known infectious diseases, such as smallpox or plague, to flourish. Indeed, it was probably Pizarro (the Spanish conquistador), on his preliminary visit to the Inca Empire, when he and his men briefly stopped at Tumbes in Peru, that smallpox was introduced.

The epidemic raged, killing the Inca Huayna Capac (the eleventh Sapa Inca – ruler or emperor), leaving Huáscar, his son by one of his sisters, to become the Sapa Inca in Cuzco. However, another son, Atahuallpa, by Huayna Capac's favourite concubine, also claimed the throne. Atahuallpa had been made Governor of Quito, administering the northern part of the empire. Huáscar alienated the nobles in an attempt to raise additional revenues, a disastrous move, as they changed their allegiance to support Atahuallpa. War broke out between the two brothers and Atahuallpa was victorious.

Although by 1531, when Pizarro returned, the war was over, the Inca empire was still weakened, and this made Pizarro's conquest easier, once he had treacherously captured the Sapa Inca. The Spaniards were noticeably immune from further outbreaks of smallpox that subsequently devastated the population, due to having contracted the illness in childhood, a fact that did not go unnoticed by the Incas, and gave the Spaniards god-like status.

It had been the gold that had attracted the Spaniards, but it was sugar that subsequently became the most lucrative commodity. This was partly because the local population had been devastated by European diseases such as measles, rubella, influenza and scarlet fever, and their consequent inability to be effective labourers required that African slaves be brought over to work the plantations. Invariably they brought their diseases with them, and as well as those mentioned in Chapter 7, there were also the vector-borne diseases of malaria and yellow fever.

Malaria in South America

Malaria has a persistent liver stage in the form of the disease that is caused by *Plasmodium vivax*, so it would have been easy for this to be transported by people. Also, as the female *Anopheles* mosquito must take a blood meal to develop her eggs, it would only have been a matter of time before the parasites that are liberated into the human bloodstream during feeding adapted to a local mosquito. Strangely though, this is not the form of malaria that is predominantly found in South America, but that caused by *Plasmodium falciparum*. While it would be possible for this species of malaria parasite to be transported in the semi-immune African, it would need to be present in the blood for a very long time for the local mosquitoes to become adapted to it. However, the ships that brought the slaves across from Africa were damp and dark, and were travelling within the tropics, so they would have provided suitable conditions for mosquitoes to breed. It would, therefore, seem more likely that it was the mosquito, together with its source of parasites – taking blood meals on the slaves – that was the means by which malaria was first introduced to the Americas. When these mosquitoes got to South America, they were probably outcompeted by the local species, but by then the parasite had already been transmitted to the local population.

It is very easy to associate jungle with disease, and particularly with infections such as malaria, but malaria has only been introduced comparatively recently into many parts of the Amazon jungle.

I was once working with some Venezuelan doctors among the Yanomami tribe, which extends across the border of Venezuela into Brazil. The people are hunter–gatherers (foraging horticulturalists), having lived in the Amazon jungle since before any recorded history, and although they had a fearsome reputation in the past, they have now settled down to a more peaceful way of life. One of their biggest problems was malaria and we were trying to work out the best way of minimizing the problem among them, bearing in mind their isolated way of life. Some of the missionaries told of whole groups of them dying from the disease within recent time, and it was quite clear that they had absolutely no resistance to malaria.

Both Wallace and Bates contracted malaria in the Amazon forest, but this was when they returned to a centre of population where the parasite was circulating – in the jungle where they had been for many months, they were free of the disease. Humboldt, who explored the part of the Amazon where I was working some 50 years before Wallace and Bates, never mentioned being ill with malaria. In more recent times, local people have introduced the parasite into parts of the Amazon where it was previously unknown. This is mostly due to gold mining, which has lured prospectors into the Amazon to seek their fortune.

Most of the indigenous Amazonian tribes have now been contacted so are able to get to health services, although the toll of ill health among them is still considerable. However, there are groups that have never made contact, either with missionaries or with special services set up to help indigenous peoples, so it is likely that they will die out from malaria before anything is known about them.

Yellow Fever

Another disease carried by mosquitoes that came to South America from Africa was yellow fever, which got its name from the jaundice that is produced as the main symptom of the disease. As well as the jaundice, there are haemorrhagic problems such as bleeding from the nose and gums, as well as internal bleeding, which are often the cause of death.

Differently from malaria, the organism responsible for yellow fever is an arbovirus, transmitted by mosquitoes of the genus *Aedes*. These are the black and white mosquitoes that were previously mentioned (see Fig. 4.1). The most important is *Ae. aegypti*, the final vector in a complex pattern of transmission that is illustrated in Fig. 8.1, which shows the differing cycles in Africa and South America. The disease is maintained in forest monkeys by various species of mosquitoes, and it is when humans come into contact with these monkeys that transmission takes place. In Africa, there is an intermediate cycle between the person and the original monkey-biting mosquito, generally in a cultivated rural environment, whereas in South America, the disease is acquired when workers are cutting down trees deep inside the forest. It is the late worker who has left it until the evening to return to his village who is more likely to get infected, as the canopy-inhabiting mosquitoes descend to ground level at this time. Having been fed upon by the monkey mosquito, the newly infected person, on returning to his village, becomes the source of blood for *Ae. aegypti*, and an urban cycle results.

Ae. aegypti likes to live close to humans, its preferred source of blood, so it breeds in water tanks, tin cans, coconut shells, old tyres and any other collections of water near to the house. Indeed, a major preventive strategy, not only for yellow fever but also for dengue, is to search around the house for any collections of water, especially if the black and white mosquito is noticed to be the kind that is biting. Water tanks can be covered with netting, or dragon fly larvae introduced, as these prey upon mosquitoes but do not contaminate the water.

Yellow fever was probably introduced to South America with the slaves in a similar manner to malaria. While *Ae. aegypti* is a familiar mosquito in all parts of the world, and may well have been present in South America when the disease was introduced, it is likely that it too came across in the slave ships, as it would have found all the conditions there

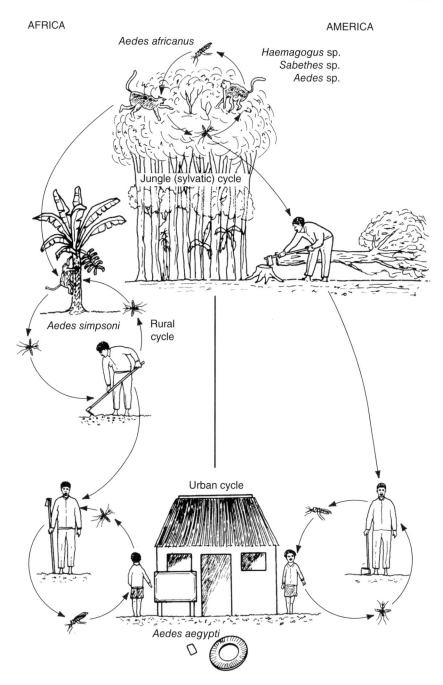

Fig. 8.1. Yellow fever transmission cycles in Africa and South America (including Panama). (From Webber, 2012, *Communicable Diseases: A Global Perspective*, 4th Edn.)

that were necessary for it to breed. Maintaining a transmission cycle on the journey over, it only needed to escape into the environment once it arrived to produce localized epidemics.

The first epidemic was in Barbados in 1647, whence it spread through other Caribbean islands and from these to ports of call in South America and the USA. Many of these subsequent epidemics were not reported in any detail, but by 1878 there was a large epidemic in the Mississippi Delta that killed 10% of the population of New Orleans and Memphis.

Alfred Russel Wallace was in South America from April 1848 until June 1852, during which time his brother, Herbert Edward Wallace came out to join him. However, Herbert only got as far as Belem, where he died in the yellow fever epidemic that was raging at that time. Alfred, who was in the interior collecting, never heard about the fate of his brother until a year later, so was not even able to be there for his funeral.

Yellow fever also disrupted the first attempt to build the Panama canal by Ferdinand de Lesseps (builder of the Suez canal) between 1881 and 1894, so it was only after pioneering work into its control had been done that the canal was finally built.

Dr Carlos Finlay, a Cuban doctor, suspected that the disease was transmitted by mosquitoes, although he was unable to prove it. This was followed up by an American bacteriologist, Walter Reed, who experimented on himself and volunteers to finally confirm that mosquitoes were the means of transmission. This opened the way to one of the first major control programmes of a vector-borne disease by Col. William C. Gorgas, who reduced the number of mosquitoes in the canal construction area to such a low level that disease transmission ceased. Work on the canal began again in 1904, opening the way to passage by ships directly between the Atlantic and Pacific in 1914.

The causative virus of yellow fever was finally isolated in 1927, and a vaccine developed that is still one of the best vaccines in the medical armoury, providing good protection for up to 10 years. Anyone entering the yellow fever areas of Africa and South America must have a valid vaccination certificate, and the authorities in Brazil have used the vaccine to protect immigrants into the Amazon by setting up vaccination stations on all roads to intercept any traffic. Despite the effectiveness of the vaccine, unlike smallpox, yellow fever can never be eradicated, because it is maintained in the wild monkey population.

Chagas' Disease

Before leaving South America, mention should be made of one disease that is indigenous to this part of the world, because it is found nowhere else. This is American trypanasomiasis, which is more commonly known as Chagas' disease (after the Brazilian physician Carlos Chagas, who described the pathogen and the disease in 1909). The disease is found throughout Central and South America, and considerable strides have been made to eradicate it from most of the area, but it may well have influenced our present state of knowledge through one of its possible early victims.

Infection is acquired through the bite of a reduvid, or kissing bug, from its habit of biting its victim at night, often on the mouth, as so well described by Charles Darwin in his account of the *Voyage of the Beagle*. The ship had anchored in Valparaiso for some time, so Darwin took the opportunity to cross the Andes to Mendoza in Argentina, as he recorded:

> We slept in the village, which is a small place surrounded by gardens, and forms the most southern part, that is cultivated, of the province of Mendoza; it is 5 leagues south of the capital. At night I experienced an attack (for it deserves no less a name) of the *Benchuca*, a species of Reduvius, the great black bug of the Pampas. It is most disgusting to feel soft wingless insects, about an inch long, crawling over one's body. Before sucking they are quite thin, but afterwards become round and bloated with blood, and in this state they are easily crushed.

The main pathology produced by infection are an enlargement of the heart, oesophagus and colon, producing symptoms very similar to those described by Darwin in letters he wrote to his friends. He suffered from chronic illness for the rest of his life, which probably contributed to him never travelling again, instead spending nearly all his time at Down House in Kent researching and putting together his great theory. The final impetus for him to publish came from the paper suggesting the same idea, sent to him by Alfred Russel Wallace, by then in Halmahera, now part of Indonesia. He had, however, amassed a vast amount of information in his self-imposed exile, making it easier for him to present to the world the theory of evolution that has had such a profound effect.

Whether Darwin did in fact suffer from Chagas' Disease will never be known, as a request to the authorities of Westminster Abbey, where he is buried, to allow DNA analysis of his remains was refused.

A Glass of Water 9

Cholera

It was just a glass of water that ended the life of one of the greatest Russian composers, Tchaikovsky...or was it? He died in 1893, reputedly from cholera, but mystery surrounds the exact nature of his death as at the time he was accused of a romantic association with a male member of the imperial family. Drinking a glass of unboiled water in the midst of a cholera epidemic was almost as certain a means of death as the poison he might have been persuaded to take in order to avoid a scandal.

The first pandemic of cholera started in 1817 in Bengal, and in the following year, it was carried to Arabia by pilgrims from Bombay who were attending the Haj. From there, it travelled as far as China and Japan across Asia, and then to East Africa with returning pilgrims from Mecca, before dying out in 1824. During the second pandemic, from 1826 to 1832, the disease reached Europe as well as travelling across the Atlantic with Irish immigrants. The third pandemic, from 1852 to 1859, was particularly severe in the USA. The disease reached South America in the 1881–1896 pandemic. This was the same pandemic that raged in Russia, the worst of the 21 countries affected. Between 14 May 1892 and 11 February 1896, there were 504,924 cases in Russia, of which 226,940 died, giving a death rate of 44.9%.

By the time cholera reached Russia, the detective work of John Snow (described below) had shown an association of the disease with contaminated water, so the Russian health authorities had issued orders that all water served in restaurants must be boiled. Unfortunately for Tchaikovsky, the restaurant where he was taking his meal had run out of boiled water, so he asked for a glass of unboiled water, saying to his friends that he had no fear of contracting the infection. By the next day, he was already complaining of an upset stomach and 3 days later had all the symptoms of cholera. Two doctors certified that he had died from cholera, although his symptoms could, to a certain extent, also have been explained by arsenic poisoning. However, Tsar Alexander III paid for his funeral and ordered that it should be in Kazan Cathedral in St Petersburg, which was the highest honour that he could be paid. The final proof would be to test the coffin contents, as arsenic remains in the body for a considerable length of time, but so far this has not been done.

The symptoms of cholera and cause of death are simple: there is such an outpouring of fluid from the bowel that the person dies from dehydration. The fluid is not diarrhoea as such, because the excreta contain no faecal material; rather, is flecked with mucus, giving it an appearance best described as looking like rice water. This is because the causative organism, *Vibrio cholerae*, binds to the cells of the intestine to produce an enterotoxin which activates an intracellular enzyme (adenyl cyclase) to move fluid from the plasma to the intestinal lumen. Large quantities of low-protein fluid, bicarbonate and potassium escape through an essentially undamaged intestine, a mechanism engineered by the cholera vibrio to flush out the normal gut flora with which it is in competition. This mechanism also provides the method for large numbers of *V. cholerae* to be excreted into the environment and thereby to continue disease transmission.

Theoretically, the treatment is straightforward: to replace the fluid loss in sufficient quantity and consistency until the body has had time to overcome the organism and the enterotoxin. This strategy, however, is the problem. In hospitals where electrolytes can be monitored, it is a simple matter to replace the fluid in sufficient quantity (gauged by the amount excreted), and fortified with the salts and other substances that are lost, to have an almost 100% recovery rate. Fluid is initially given by intravenous infusion, and then, as the person recovers, it can be replaced by oral fluids containing the missing ingredients, which are known as oral rehydration solutions (ORS). But in many parts of the world, or in the circumstances of an epidemic, electrolytes cannot be monitored, and even though the person might receive sufficient fluid, the essential salts are missing.

In the face of an epidemic it is generally better to set up treatment centres rather than to flood the hospital(s) with patients, which could spread infection to those who are already ill and compromise the normal hospital services. These centres can be schools, churches, warehouses or similar places, and in one location I even came across a large mango tree with bottles of intravenous fluid hanging from its branches, as there was nowhere else to treat everybody.

Cholera is nearly always transmitted by water, and the health authorities in St Petersburg had made good regulations to control the epidemic of 1892, but the reason these were not effective was because of a very divided society – the rich upper class for which the regulations were effective, and the vast majority of the impoverished population who probably had little to cook with, let alone set aside a valuable cooking pot of boiled water. Indeed, cholera became regarded as a disease of the poor, and this was one of the factors that led to the development of a conspiracy theory over the death of Tchaikovsky. The aristocracy could not accept that the great composer had died from a disease so associated with the lower classes.

Even without knowing the causative organism, the epidemiology of the disease was worked out by John Snow (1813–1858), a London doctor, in 1854. Epidemiology, the science of the causative factors of a disease, is based on three simple concepts that can be summarized as persons, place and time. The main theory at that time was miasma, or bad smell, which actually had certain aspects of truth because cholera was associated with contaminated (smelly) water, as Snow was to demonstrate. But this was the problem – because of the similarity between the smell itself and the smelly water, it took a lot of evidence to prove the real cause.

Snow first recorded the water company from which people were supplied with water and found that there were more cases of cholera in users of the water supplier that had an inlet downstream to the sewage outflow. He then made a more detailed study of an outbreak in Soho and found a strong association with people who took their water from the well in Broad Street. In addition, he was particularly interested in a case of cholera in a wealthy lady in Highgate that seemed to be an exception. However, he discovered that because the lady had once lived in Soho, she took a particular liking to the taste of the water from the Broad Street Well and used to send her maid to collect water for her, a fatal tipple. Snow famously brought the epidemic to an end by persuading the authorities to remove the handle of the Broad Street Pump and is ironically commemorated in his action, where the old Broad Street used to be, by a pub, despite being a teetotaller.

Over a century later, I was faced with investigating an epidemic of cholera in Tanzania which had all the same features of trying to convince the local authorities of the real cause. Like the first pandemic of cholera, but this time caused by a new biotype known as El Tor (after the quarantine station in Sinai from which it was first isolated in 1906), this new epidemic came to East Africa with a pilgrim returning from the Haj. When the person died, the body was carefully cleaned, including evacuation of the bowel contents, as was the practice in the Islamic religion. Not surprisingly, a few days later, some of the attendants that had been responsible for preparing the body developed cholera, and the epidemic soon started. It took the investigators some time to realize how the epidemic was being spread, but once they understood that it was the burial practice, this was banned. The epidemic had already spread to other parts of Tanzania, including the south-west of the country, where I had recently arrived. Before I came, the authorities had not only banned the Islamic burial practice, despite this part of the country being predominantly Christian, but also banned the consumption of fish because the epidemic was centred on the northern shores of Lake Nyasa (known as Lake Malawi by other countries). This second ban was based on the finding of cholera vibrios in the intestines of fish caught from the lake by a visiting microbiologist.

Roadblocks had been erected to prevent the transport of fish from the lake, so depriving the people of their main export and local food source. It seemed that the cholera epidemic might soon be replaced by malnutrition in children.

I did not agree with the fish ban and set about using the epidemiological principles developed by Snow. I found that it was predominantly adult women living in villages along the rivers that ran into the lake, rather than those in the lake villages where the fish were caught, that were contracting cholera. It was quite easy to see from the way the people cooked the fish, by putting them on a fire until the skin was completely burnt, that even if they had been infected with vibrios, these could not have survived this incineration. My conclusion was that it was the women, who were the collectors of water, who in order to reduce the amount of water that they needed to carry back to their houses, had drunk their fill from the places in the rivers where water was taken from. Like the advice in St Petersburg, I recommended that all drinking water was boiled, and the ban on fish lifted, but my advice was not taken and the epidemic continued.

Fortuitously for me, but not for those that were suffering, another epidemic soon broke out on Lake Rukwa, in another part of Tanzania. Here the cases were in villages along the lake shore, whose inhabitants equally consumed fish; some villages had no cholera, while in others many succumbed, the main difference being that the cholera-free villages had piped water supplies. Even more conclusive was one particular river, where the third parameter of time was particularly valuable. By plotting the date when the first cases occurred in villages along the side of the river, it was clear that the upper villages were the first to get the infection, followed by those lower down in a sequential fashion. This was because latrines had been built too close to the river, so when cases developed in a village, it was the one downstream from it that was next to suffer, and each time the river water was contaminated by sewage seepage.

Convinced this time, the authorities did agree with my findings and replaced the fish ban with an instruction to boil drinking water. Fortunately Tanzania has a very good system of village health committees, so it was possible to check that families had the means to boil their water and were doing so. This time, the epidemic did come to an end.

There would not have been an epidemic in the first place if everybody had been able to obtain their water from a safe water supply, which is one of the main methods of improving health in developing countries. Cholera comes in epidemic form and causes panic, but ordinary diarrhoeal diseases are present for much of the time and account for a far larger number of deaths in children, many of which could be prevented by proper water supplies.

Ewald has hypothesized that cholera originated in the Harappan or Indus Valley civilization, which flourished in what is now Pakistan from 2500 to 1700 BC. Ironically, these people had a very advanced system of water supply and drainage that used brick-lined culverts, but the area was liable to flooding, and excavations have revealed signs of several major floods. These would have contaminated the water supply, and if cholera had been introduced into the area, it could have had a devastating effect and help to explain why the civilization came to such a sudden end. (Perversely, the main reason that is believed to have caused the demise of Mohenjo Daro, the main city of the civilization, was the disappearing water supply due to the river changing its course.)

Cholera organisms are found in the environment, where they exist in a natural cycle in copepods and other zooplankton as non-agglutinable (or non-cholera) vibrios. These are known to mutate, with shifts from the non-agglutinable to the glutinable form, and if such a transformation had coincided with a flood, then a cholera epidemic would have developed. It was, however, a very long time from the Indus Valley civilization until the first cholera pandemic of 1817, and it seems likely that there would have been recorded outbreaks before then if that civilization had been the origin.

Typhoid

It was possibly another glass of water that led to the death of Queen Victoria's husband and almost destroyed the British monarchy, as the bereaved Queen turned in on herself to become a recluse in her Scottish castle. In the hills near Balmoral, there is a well called the Prince's Well, in honour of Prince Albert (Fig. 9.1). He had probably visited it many times and partaken of its water, but it was shortly after his last visit to the well that he contracted typhoid. Whether the well was the source of the typhoid – an unlucky contamination of a probably good source of water – or whether the infection was from some other place cannot be determined, although it was not long after visiting the well that he became ill.

John Snow, who had worked out the epidemiology of cholera, was actually an anaesthetist and one of the first people to use chloroform. He had administered chloroform to a grateful Queen for the last two of her deliveries, as she hated the pain of childbirth. Fortunately, he was as careful with his anaesthetics as he was with his investigations into the cause of cholera, as the margin of safety with chloroform is a narrow one, and when it subsequently became more frequently used, there were several deaths. It would, therefore, seem almost certain that the Queen would have known about the water transmission of cholera, and Snow would have advised the royal household that all drinking water should be boiled. So you can imagine the scene at the Prince's Well, where a gallant Albert asks for a glass of water, while a more cautious Queen tells him that it has not been boiled: 'But my dear, it is pure highland water', replies Albert. It probably was on most occasions, but it could have been contaminated on this one.

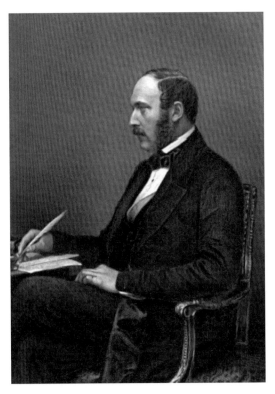

Fig. 9.1. Prince Albert, whose death from typhoid threatened the future of the British Monarchy. (After a photograph taken by John Jabez Edwin Mayall, 1860, public domain.)

Typhoid is often given the more useful description of typhoid fever, because it is the fever that is the predominant feature of the disease. This rises in a stepwise fashion to a crisis, from which the patient either survives or dies. Unlike the cholera vibrio, the causative organism of typhoid attacks the bowel, producing ulceration, and also invades the gall bladder, where it can remain for many years. This leads to the carrier state, where a person who has recovered from the infection can cause epidemics by contaminating food or water if they are not particularly careful with their personal hygiene. Such people remain carriers for many years – as long as 50 years – and one of the most famous was nicknamed 'Typhoid Mary' for the number of epidemics she caused over the period of her life.

In slums and many developing countries, typhoid circulates in the community and children develop a certain degree of immunity, but if a stranger should enter into the neighbourhood, then they are likely to contract the disease. This is because typhoid is one of the diseases that is dose dependent, so that when there are low doses of infecting organisms, infection may not occur, but even in those with some immunity a high dose of organisms will cause the disease. There are both oral and inject-able vaccines, which offer a good deal of protection, but if the immunized person is unfortunate enough to swallow a large dose of organisms, they may still get the disease.

The organism responsible for typhoid belongs to the group of organ-isms called *Salmonella*. A less serious form of the disease, also caused by a *Salmonella*, is paratyphoid, while other members of the group are respon-sible for food poisoning, which is covered in Chapter 15.

Prevention

When investigating the cholera epidemics, the only precaution I took was to boil my drinking water and prepare my own food, simple things that could have been done by anybody. It is often public health measures that are all that is required to prevent disease with, in the case of typhoid and several other diseases, reinforcement by vaccination.

The Great War **10**

It was to be the 'war that ends all wars', which sadly it was not, but in many ways the 1914–1918 global conflict was to change many aspects of life. In the realm of combat, it was the last war in which armies of men fought each other, as it saw the birth of aerial warfare. After this, the killing and carnage would involve the rest of the population. No longer would war mean the killing of a nation's young men, but women and children as well, and often in greater numbers than active combatants.

It was near the Latin Bridge in Sarajevo that the event that would start World War I took place. Archduke Franz Ferdinand, the crown prince of the Austro–Hungarian Empire, and his wife Sophie had come to Serbia on a goodwill visit. While they were driving along Hamidije Kreševljakovića, a bomb was thrown at their vehicle, killing bodyguards and bystanders but missing the royal couple. The police and security officers tried to persuade the Archduke to take shelter in case there was another attempt, but he insisted on continuing with the motorcade – it was important that he convey the message of peace and understanding that he had come to deliver. Unfortunately, the driver turned the wrong way at a T-junction, going towards the Latin Bridge instead of away from it. When he realized his mistake he attempted to reverse the car but, coincidentally, one of the assassins, Gavrilo Princip, having escaped from the foiled bomb attempt, found himself right next to the now stationary vehicle. Nervously, he took out his revolver and with just two shots killed both the Archduke and Sophie. Serbia was blamed for the killings and, a month later, a war-eager Germany began the conflict.

Not only did a driver's mistake start World War I but, inadvertently, World War II as well, because the Great War had a huge effect on Germany's future leader. Reduced to trench warfare, the battle lines of World War I moved backwards and forwards across the devastated fields of Belgium. Huge battles such as the Somme, with considerable loss of life, would push the battle lines back against the Germans, only to be retaken a few months later, and return to much as they were. By 1918, an exhausted

Germany, faced by the arrival of American troops and an escalation of the conflict that it knew it could not sustain, made one last major attack. At first this seemed to be achieving its objective: the Allies were pushed back, and to the soldier in the trench it looked as if Germany was about to win, when quite suddenly the advance ceased and peace was made. Among those serving in the trenches was Adolf Hitler. Embittered by the collapse of the German High Command and the terms of the peace agreement – a grudge he carried with him for the rest of his life – when the time came and he had risen to power, much of the reason for another war was revenge for what had happened.

For the countries that took part in World War I, the loss of human life was enormous, and it had not just been losses of professional soldiers, but of conscripts as well. These were in such numbers that nearly the entire workforce was signed up and the demography of the country changed. One only needs to look at the war memorials that stand in every village in the UK to realize the implications that this change had. Sometimes the numbers killed were so great that the village literally disappeared, while in others it was so severely compromised that it never recovered its former size. Estates collapsed, the farming system changed, wives lost their husbands and young women their future marriage partners.

Yet despite this loss of men, soon after the war had finished, an even greater loss of life, and this time cutting right across all ages and both sexes, was to take place: from influenza. The 1918 pandemic is estimated to have infected 50% of the world's population, half of whom probably did not have a severe enough infection to require medical attention. It is thought that some 20–40 million were killed, of which 600,000 died in the USA and 200,000 in England and Wales. Case fatality rates in countries in Africa and the Indian subcontinent were much higher owing to the state of nutrition and lack of treatment of complications. In some populations, such as those in Alaska and the Pacific Islands, and the indigenous peoples of Australia and New Zealand, extremely high death rates were recorded. Entire villages were wiped out and some populations never properly recovered.

There has been much speculation as to why this epidemic was so severe, even leading to attempts to reproduce the virus from post-mortem material that survives from that time. While this might shed some light on the problem, the other aspect to be considered is the host response to the virus. Unlike previous pandemics, there is evidence of an aberrant host response, which caused extensive damage in the lungs, particularly affecting the 20–40-year age group. This might have been due to some sort of sensitivity from previous exposure to recent strains of influenza, as there were several waves of infection one after another, rather similar to what can happen in dengue. Fortunately, it does seem to have been a unique event, as such a severe reaction has not occurred again.

Dengue is an arboviral disease spread by members of the *Aedes* family of mosquitoes (Fig. 4.1.), presenting as a fever with headache and pains in the joints, which give it the alternative name of break-bone disease. Originally, it was a mild infection rather like influenza, with which it was often initially confused, but in the 1960s a more severe form called dengue haemorrhagic fever (DHF) was reported from Thailand. As its name suggests, there was bleeding into the skin and tissues, which produced shock and deaths from this normally non-fatal disease. There are four dengue viruses, and it is thought that DHF is due to sensitization with another dengue serotype from a previous infection, type 2 being the most potent. Although this sensitization results in haemorrhagic symptoms in DHF, a similar type of sensitization may have taken place during the waves of influenza that occurred close together in the 1918–1920 pandemic.

Influenza comes in epidemics, and there have been many over the centuries. The first recognized epidemic started in Asia in 1580 and spread to Europe, Africa and even North America. The first pandemic was from 1729 to 1733, originating in Russia and spreading to the rest of the world in the following years, producing a high death rate. The second originated in China in 1781 and infected 10 million people worldwide by the following year but, luckily, the death rate was low. China and Russia then took alternate turns, with China being the origin of the 1830–1833 pandemic and Russia of the 1889–1892 pandemic. The latter is probably the first pandemic that can be described as truly global, and some 300,000 are thought to have died during it. The final pandemic of the 19th century was from 1898 to 1900, but this was mainly mild and experience of it probably protected older people in subsequent epidemics.

There are three types of the influenza virus, A, B and C, with the last being responsible for mild infections and B less serious than A. When the A virus is examined with an electron microscope, spikes can be seen that are formed from a surface protein haemagglutinin (HA) and from a neuramidase (NA), which have led to the development of several subtypes (H1N1, H2N2, H3N2, etc.). Birds, especially aquatic birds, form the natural reservoir of all known influenza A subtypes, but they are also found in pigs, horses and other animals. Pigs in particular are receptors for both the avian and human viruses, between which a reassortment can take place, leading to new strains of the virus that are liable to result in pandemic spread. However, the most severe form of influenza known, the A/H1N1 of 1918, is thought to have infected humans directly from aquatic birds. This was a novel influenza virus, to which the general population had no immunity and so it was able to spread from person to person.

As most of the world was involved in World War I, events of the conflict dominated the news in those countries. Spain, being neutral, was not so encumbered, so when the epidemic of flu broke out there it became headline news and was called the Spanish flu. The flu did not originate in Spain though, and outbreaks were reported simultaneously in three US prisons (in Detroit in Michigan, San Quentin in California, and also in South Carolina) during March 1918. From these areas it was carried by American troops going to battlefields in Europe, exacerbated by their cramped military accommodation and their general deployment. There was then a second wave in 1918–1919 and a third in 1919–1920, in which a more virulent form of infection occurred. This particularly attacked 20–40 year olds, rather than the young and the elderly, who are normally the main victims of a flu epidemic, and the 20–40 year olds were the very age group most required to rebuild nations after the devastation of the war.

With three outbreaks having occurred almost simultaneously in US prisons, it would seem that there must have been a single initiating case, and this has been traced to Chinese labourers working in the prisons. There was considerable emigration from China at that time, and while it cannot be shown conclusively, knowing what has happened in subsequent outbreaks, it would seem that China might well have been the origin of the 1918 pandemic, as it had been of those in earlier centuries.

The next flu pandemic, called the Asian flu, started in Yunnan Province, China, in February 1957. It was of the A/H2N2 type and was considered to be a reassortment of the human and avian viruses, probably brought about by an intermediate mammalian host, most likely a pig. It rapidly spread throughout the world, mainly along shipping routes, while in Europe outbreaks coincided with the start of the autumn school term, as many of us that were infected may remember. My school just died, as there was nobody around – no pupils to attend the classes and no teachers to instruct them. As one of the few still wandering around, it was an eerie experience. I must also have been infected but, by some good fortune, was not confined to my bed. Instead, I was alone in an empty school.

In the UK cases were concentrated in schoolchildren, although the greatest mortality was in the elderly and pregnant women. This was a new risk group and, even though pregnant women are not generally more susceptible, with some of the strains of flu they do need extra protection.

The next pandemic in 1968 also started in China, with a particularly large number of cases in Hong Kong (then a British colony), so it was called the Hong Kong flu. It probably had a similar origin to the 1957 pandemic in being a reassortment of avian and human viruses. Like the previous pandemic, it did not have the high mortality of the 1918 epidemic, and this was thought to be due to previous exposure to similar virus for some groups of the population. This happened because the causative virus was a mixture of avian and human viruses, rather than a pure avian strain, as probably occurred in 1918. Overall, there were estimated to be 3 million fatalities and an overall case fatality rate of 0.5%.

There was another global outbreak in 1977, the so-called 'Russian flu', but here again, this had previously been detected in three Chinese provinces. Russia has a long border with China, and this might well have been the reason that historical epidemics were thought to have originated in Russia rather than China. The 1977 outbreak did not have all the features of a pandemic, affecting mainly people under 20 years of age, indicating that older age groups had past experience of the virus.

Unlike most diseases, coming out of Africa, influenza seems to be an original Chinese disease, and nearly all pandemics can be traced to this origin. It is also particularly the southern provinces of China that are responsible, those that enjoy a culinary custom of eating a large range of animals, kept alive in cages or fish tanks, until they are ready for the table. Conditions are primitive and the general state of hygiene poor, allowing ample opportunity for the transfer of infection from animals to humans, should this be a possibility. (This is covered in more detail in Chapter 12.) Ducks and pigs have been domesticated for some 9500 years, and are particularly common items of food in this part of the world. Indeed, the pig is used like a food-waste recycling plant, kept in a cage next to the house and fed food remains. When it is of a sufficient size it is killed for the table and another put in its place, with probably its first meal the remains of its predecessor.

The outbreak of avian influenza (A/H5N1) in 2003 raised considerable concern because it gave many indications that it could become like the devastating epidemic of 1918. It first started in Hong Kong in 1997, when avian influenza devastated the domestic fowl population, but there were also 18 human cases (six of which died). The same virus was identified in fowl in 2002, resulting in mass slaughter of chickens, but despite these draconian measures there were four more cases in humans, all of which died. In 2003, human cases were identified in China and Vietnam, in all involving some 400 people, with a 60% mortality. Fortunately, close contact with fowl seemed to be required to become infected. However, should a reassortment take place with a human influenza strain, this could make transmission easier, with devastating consequences. So far this has not happened, and progress has been made in preparing a vaccine against A/H5N1, but there are still all the problems of manufacturing enough vaccine and administering it to sufficient people to halt a pandemic.

While waterbirds are the natural reservoir of influenza virus, it does not affect them and has remained unchanged in its genetic sequence for the past 85 years. The birds show no symptoms, the virus being limited to the intestinal tissues, though it can of course be passed in their excreta. This is thought to be how infection starts, perhaps with wild ducks mixing with domestic ones, but such are the migratory patterns and huge numbers of wild waterfowl that nothing can be done to control infection developing in this way. However, the conditions in southern China in which people live in close proximity with poultry and animals, often in cramped and unhygienic conditions, offer an ideal environment for transmission. This is probably how new strains of influenza originated in the past and might well do in the future, so it is hoped that by then prevention will have been implemented and the likelihood of future outbreaks thereby reduced.

Man's Best Friend?   **11**

Rabies

The dog probably domesticated itself, realizing that there were benefits in hanging around human settlements where there would have been odd scraps of food, and particularly bones, that it could eat. As men went off on hunting parties they were probably trailed by wolves, which in time they found could be useful in assisting the hunt, and by barking to warn of danger back in the home. Gradually, this association became accepted, and wolves were welcomed into the settlement and actively fed. This probably occurred some 14,000 to 12,000 years ago, meaning that members of the dog family are man's oldest domesticated animal.

This long association has allowed humans plenty of time to contract the diseases of dogs or for them to serve as reservoirs of an intermediate infection, as can be seen in Table 11.1. After humans, no other animal poses such a risk in the number and kind of disease that it can transmit to us. Some of these have already been mentioned, such as plague, typhus, Chagas' disease and schistosomiasis in which the dog plays an indirect part, but of more direct involvement are rabies, hydatid disease and toxacariasis.

There is no cure for established rabies and it must be one of the worst forms of death there can be. Although it starts off mild, with fever, sore throat and loss of appetite, it then enters the excitable stage, in which the person has difficulty in swallowing and becomes anxious – you can see the terror written across their face. The classic symptom is of hydrophobia (fear of water), in which the person shows panic when presented with liquids, but then cannot drink them owing to difficulty in swallowing. There is an increase in salivation, so the person shows frothing at the mouth. Generalized convulsions ensue, with the unfortunate victim dying from convulsions or progressive paralysis.

The first terminal case I saw was in an African child, bitten by a young dog it had been playing with. Sadly, it is children who are the most common victims and, as so often happens, as in this case, children of a

Table 11.1. Infections transmitted to humans from dogs and cats or in which the dog or cat is the reservoir. (From Webber, 2012, *Communicable Diseases: A Global Perspective*, 4th Edn.)

Organism	Dogs	Cats
Viruses	Arboviruses	
	Nipah	Nipah
	Rabies	Rabies
Bacteria	Anthrax	Anthrax
	Brucella canis	*Bartonella benselae* (cat-scratch disease)
	Clostridium tetani	*Chlamydia psittaci* (conjunctivitis)
	Campylobacter jejuni	*Campylobacter jejuni*
	Capnocytophaga	
	Escherichia coli	
	Leptospira canicola	
	Mycobacterium	
	Pasteurellosis	
	Salmonella	*Salmonella*
	Spirium minus	
	Tularaemia	
	Yersinia pestis (plague)	*Yersinia pestis*
Rickettsiae	*Coxiella burnetii* (Q fever)	*Coxiella burnetii*
	Rickettsia rickettsii, R. conorii, R. africae, R. australis, R. siberica, R. typhi (murine typhus)	*Rickettsia typhi*
Fungi	Dermatophytosis (tinea)	Dermatophytosis (tinea)
	Microsporum canis	*Microsporum canis*
		Sporothrix schenkii
Protozoa	Chagas' disease	
	Cryptosporidiosis	Cryptosporidiosis
	Isospora belli	*Isospora belli*
	Leishmaniasis	*Toxoplasma gondii*
Helminths	*Ancylostoma braziliense, A. caninum, A. ceylonicum* (larva migrans)	*Ancylostoma braziliense, A. caninum, A. ceylonicum*
	Brugia malayi, B. pahangi, B. patei	*Brugia malayi, B. pahangi, B. patei*
	Capillaria aerophilia	*Capillaria aerophilia*
	Diphylobothrium latum	*Diphylobothrium latum*
	Dipylidium canium	
	Dirofilaria immitis, D. repens	*Dirofilaria immitis, D. repens*
	Dracunculus medinensis	
	Echinococcus granulosus, E. multilocularis, E. vogeli	
	Echinostoma	

Continued

Table 11.1. Continued.

Organism	Dogs	Cats
	Gnathostoma spinigerum	*Gnathostoma spinigerum*
	Heterophyes heterophyes	*Heterophyes heterophyes*
	Metagonimus yokagawi	*Metagonimus yokagawi*
	Multiceps multiceps	
	Clonorchis sinensis	*Clonorchis sinensis*
	Opisthorchis felineus, O. viverrini	*Opisthorchis felineus, O. viverrini*
	Paragonimus westermani,	*Paragonimus westermani,*
	P. africanus, P. calensis,	*P. africanus, P. calensis,*
	P. heterotremus, P. kellicotti,	*P. heterotremus,*
	P. mexicanus, P. philippinensis,	*P. kellicotti, P. mexicanus,*
	P. polonaise, P. uterobilateralis	*P. philippensis,*
		P. polonaise,
		P. uterobilateralis
	Schistosoma japonicum	*Schistosoma japonicum*
	Strongyloides stercoralis	*Strongyloides stercoralis*
	Toxocara canis	*Toxocara cati*
	Trichinella spiralis	*Trichinella spiralis*
Arthropods	Fleas	Fleas
	Pentastomids (*Linguatula*)	
	Ticks	

family play together, so the same rabid dog went round and bit all the children. The parents had lost all their children in one tragic and distressing episode.

While there is a vaccine available, it is beyond the reach of many, and in the case of children their parents might not realize what had happened, so they might not take the necessary action. Rabies is common in Russia, Africa, Asia and South America. It is estimated that there are 24,000 deaths per annum in Africa and a further 20,000 in India alone. Cases in India are increasing as a result of a parliamentary act, passed in 2001, outlawing the killing of dogs. After India, Vietnam, followed by Thailand, are the most infected countries. Male children seem to be more vulnerable than female children.

While in most diseases vaccination needs to be given in advance for the body to develop an immune response, quite remarkably in rabies, post-exposure vaccination is possible. Louis Pasteur, inspired by Jenner's earlier contribution (and honouring his work by coining the term *vaccine*), set about investigating vaccination.

The rabies vaccine was actually developed by Emile Roux, a colleague of Pasteur, and had only been tried out on dogs, but Pasteur took the risk of giving it to 9-year-old Joseph Meister, who had been badly mauled by a rabid dog, on 6 July 1885. Not only had it not been tried on humans before, but Pasteur was not a registered physician, so he took a double risk. Because of the fear of rabies circulating at that time, when the person bitten by a rabid dog could be killed or driven to commit suicide, he decided to try to save the boy's life. Fortunately for him and the world, it was a success and the boy survived.

The present-day versions of the rabies vaccine are cell-culture-based vaccines, much improved from earlier vaccines, which contained animal products that could cause serious reactions. There is, however, still some risk, so routine vaccination is normally only given to people who could get infected, such as veterinary surgeons and animal handlers. For tourists and visitors entering a rabies area, the general advice is that they do not need to have pre-exposure vaccination unless they are likely to be unable to reach a vaccination centre within 24 hours. This is the length of time within which post-exposure vaccination can be effectively given.

Other animals transmitting rabies, especially the vampire bat in South America, have engendered a level of fear out of all proportion to their importance. Most of the rabies is transmitted to cattle, in which it can be a problem, but it is very rare for humans to get infected this way. Sleeping under a mosquito net, as malaria is a more likely danger, will adequately prevent vampire bats from biting, should they be in the vicinity. It is not just vampire bats that pose a risk, though, as insectivorous and frugivorous species have been found to be infected with rabies as well. Going into caves, especially in parts of Africa, should be done with caution and at least a mask worn, as infection appears to be due to inhaling an aerosol of bat guano.

Rigid control of animals (with obligatory quarantine) has kept the UK, Australia and other countries practising these methods free of infection. All dogs should be licensed and vaccinated, and all strays destroyed.

Control of the wild animal reservoirs of rabies is a massive undertaking and their total destruction over large areas can upset the ecological balance, so vaccination is a preferable strategy. Bait laced with vaccine has been effective in much of Europe and Canada. In vampire bat areas, attempts to vaccinate in this way have been unsuccessful, but cattle can be vaccinated instead.

Hydatid Disease

Hydatid disease is one of those conditions that seems to have gained little notice by the general public, but is as serious and unpleasant as many more widely known diseases. Cysts develop in parts of the body, especially the liver, lung, abdomen, kidney and brain, in this descending order of frequency. As the cysts increase in size they cause serious problems, depending on where they are found, with infection sometimes ending fatally. The cyst contents are infective, so if they rupture accidentally or during operations to remove them, numerous new cysts are formed. The liberation of so much foreign protein into the body can result in a severe anaphylactic reaction.

The causative organism is *Echinococcus granulosus*, a tapeworm infecting members of the dog family. Eggs are passed in dog faeces and contaminate pastureland so that sheep, pigs, goats, cattle, camels and horses swallow the eggs and develop hydatid cysts inside their bodies. Essentially, the hydatid cyst is a fluid-filled sac containing enormous numbers of the head part of the adult tapeworm (called a scolex). The common means of infection is for the dog to be fed the offal of domesticated animals, from which the liberated scolex develops into an adult tapeworm.

Humans can become infected from eating fruit or vegetables contaminated by dog faeces, drinking water that has been similarly contaminated (a particular problem in the Arctic areas of Greenland and Spitsbergen) and also by close contact with dogs from touching them or being licked by them. When a dog licks itself around the anal region, it spreads eggs all over its body as well as them sticking to its tongue.

In the Turkana people, who live near the lake of that name in northern Kenya, there is a particular custom that has led to an extremely high level of infection. When the parents go out fishing or attending to their other duties, they leave their young children in the care of 'nursemaid' dogs. These have been trained to look after the infants, preventing them from straying from the household, and cleaning up the child's excreta-covered-bottom by licking it. In this way, eggs are spread all over the child's body, with the result that some are invariably swallowed and hydatid cysts develop inside them. However, there is a considerable time lag in the development of the cysts, and it is not until adulthood that they generally start to cause symptoms, so the Turkana find it difficult to accept that the cause is the nursemaid dogs.

In the colder regions of the world there is an even more unpleasant form of hydatid disease caused by *Echinococcus multilocularis*, which, as its name suggests, produces multiple lesions rather than single cysts – invading the body much in the same way as a metastatic cancer. It is found in Siberia, Alaska and northern Canada, as well as in the increasingly popular tourist areas of Spitsbergen and Greenland. Although it is a parasite of foxes and husky dogs, the greatest danger is contamination of water, so even though that stream of clear fresh Arctic water looks like the advert on some plastic bottle, do not be tempted to drink it.

In many of the danger areas of the Arctic, signs have been erected to warn people against drinking surface water, but equal precaution should be exercised when touching husky dogs as they are becoming increasingly popular with tourists. It is not just in Africa that danger from disease lurks; it is also found in the pure cold of the Arctic.

Trichinosis (caused by species of *Trichinella*, and already mentioned in Chapter 3) has an alternative cycle of transmission involving the polar bear and seal in the Arctic, with the result that polar bears can accumulate high levels of larvae encysted in their bodies. Early Arctic explorers, desperate for food, often ate polar bear meat raw, so became infected with large doses of *Trichinella*, sometimes with a fatal outcome. Originally, this was one of the candidates for the demise of everyone in the Franklin expedition of 1845; however, lead poisoning from pipes in the ship's water system, or poor-quality canned food, now seem to be the more likely cause.

Toxocariasis

Toxocariasis is perhaps a better known disease of dogs than hydatid disease, as cases of children infected in playgrounds often get reported in the press. These can result in blindness if a wandering larva of the dog roundworm *Toxocara canis* should settle in the eye, while fever, cough, rash and the involvement of other organs can also occur.

Infection is acquired by swallowing the eggs – obtained from stroking or being licked by a dog, or from soil or vegetables contaminated by dog faeces. The typical picture is of the young child playing with soil frequented by dogs, such as sandpits, and then putting their fingers in their mouths. The eggs are resistant to desiccation and remain in the soil for many months, so that soil in parks and other places where dogs are taken for walks can become heavily contaminated. It is mainly for the prevention of this disease that dog owners are required to clear up their animals' faeces.

There is also a form of this roundworm transmitted by cats, appropriately called *Toxocara cati*, but because of the more hygienic nature of cats in tending to dig a hole to bury their faeces, it is less of a problem. A more serious disease in which cats are involved, and one of the most remarkable parasite adaptations that has ever been found, is that of *Toxoplasma gondii*.

Toxoplasmosis

The infecting organism is related to the malaria parasite and is found in the intestines of cats. It undergoes a series of asexual multiplications in the epithelial cells of the intestines before sexual forms are produced to form oocysts. These are discharged in the cat faeces, where they are inadvertently ingested by many different animals, such as sheep and pigs, as well as the main prey species, the mouse. From the oocysts, toxoplasmas develop that invade many parts of the body, including the central nervous system, where small inflammatory foci (pseudocysts) are formed.

Children normally become infected when playing in sand pits that cats have used when burying their faeces, while adults often acquire infection from eating undercooked mutton or pork. There is a particularly high incidence of the disease in France, with the predilection of the French for eating semi-raw meat in their search for new culinary experiences.

Like dogs, cats lick their fur and, while washing themselves around the anal region, pick up oocysts. These are scattered all over their bodies, to be picked up by anybody stroking a cat. This is one of the many reasons why it is so important to wash one's hands before eating and not to feed pets at meal times.

Infection is surprisingly common, and in some countries up to 40% of the population show seropositivity to having come in contact with the disease. It was, therefore, assumed for some time that only recent infection in a pregnant woman, especially in the first 3 months of her pregnancy, was the only serious consequence. The developing fetus is affected by damage to several organs, especially the liver, eye and brain. Both hydrocephaly (a large head produced by excess fluid in the brain) and microcephaly (a small head and associated incomplete brain development) can result, and if too many organs are involved, the infant will not survive.

While this is a tragic result for the infant and its parents, it does only affect a minority. But as pseudocysts are formed in many parts of the body, including the brain, might they not produce more damage than the mild fever and enlarged lymph nodes that can result from infection?

The main prey of the cat is the mouse, which can easily become infected from consuming food contaminated by cat excrement, or indirectly from an aerosol of organisms produced from dried faeces. When pseudocysts develop in the brain of the mouse, they actually encourage its capture by reducing its reaction time. The mouse becomes slower at taking avoiding action and so is more easily caught by the cat. This really must be one of the cleverest adaptations by a parasite to ensure its continued transmission.

So, transferring this finding to humans, it has been suggested that infection with toxoplasmosis could similarly reduce reaction time and make us less quick at taking avoiding action. This could be relevant to road traffic accidents, either for the pedestrian about to step off a pavement into the path of an oncoming car, or for the driver when faced with a dangerous situation. It could also have implications in a number of other work-related accidents involving machine tools. It is difficult to test this proposition because reaction time changes with age and a number of other factors, but it would seem that there is a possibility that toxoplasmosis has wider implications than just for the woman in early pregnancy.

Beef and Pork Tapeworms

Being eaten is probably one of the most ancient methods by which parasites have been transmitted. It was the hunter or scavenger human that lived on the carcases of dead animals that would have acquired some infections this way, but when the pig was domesticated in China in 7500 BC and the cow by the Indus Valley civilization in about 7000 BC, infecting people with parasites became easier. Most of the diseases transmitted to humans by the two commonest food animals, cattle and pigs, are listed in Table 11.2.

Table 11.2. Infections transmitted to humans from cattle and pigs or in which cattle and pigs are the reservoir. (From Webber, 2012, *Communicable Diseases: A Global Perspective*, 4th Edn.)

Organism	Cattle	Pigs
Viruses	Cowpox	Avian influenza
	Crimean–Congo haemorrhagic fever	Crimean–Congo haemorrhagic fever
		Influenza
	Hepatitis E	Hepatitis E
	Rabies	Japanese encephalitis
	Rift Valley fever	La Crosse encephalitis
		Manangle
		Nipah
		Severe acute respiratory syndrome (SARS)
Prion	Creutzfeldt–Jakob (variant)	
Bacteria	Anthrax	Anthrax
	Brucella abortus	*Brucella suis*, *B. melitensis*, *B. abortus*
	Campylobacter jejuni	*Campylobacter jejuni*
	Clostridium perfringens	*Clostridium perfringens*
	Escherichia coli O157	
	Leptospira interrogans Hardjo	*Leptospira interrogans* Pomona
	Lyme disease	
	Mycobacterium bovis	
	Salmonella	*Salmonella*
	Staphylococcal food poisoning	
	Streptococcal infection	Yersiniosis
	Tetanus	Tetanus
Rickettsia	Q fever	
Fungi	Coccidioidomycosis	Coccidioidomycosis
	Cryptococcosis	
	Trichophyton verrucosum	
Protozoa	Babesiosis	*Balantidium coli*
	Cryptosporidiosis	Cryptosporidiosis
	Toxoplasmosis	Toxoplasmosis
		Trypanosoma brucei gambiense
Helminths	*Fasciola hepatica*	
	Fasciolopsis buski	*Fasciolopsis buski*
		Heterophyes heterophyes
		Metagonimus yokogawai
		Clonorchis sinensis
		Opisthorchis viverrini
		Paragonimus westermani, *P. africanus*, *P. calensis*, *P. heterotremus*, *P. kellicotti*, *P. mexicanus*, *P. philippinensis*, *P. pulmonalis*, *P. uterobilateralis*

Continued

Table 11.2. Continued.

Organism	Cattle	Pigs
	Schistosoma japonicum	*Schistosoma japonicum*
	Taenia saginata	*Taenia solium*
		Trichinella spiralis, *T. nelsoni*,
		T. nativea
Arthropods	Pentastomids (*Linguatula*)	
	Ticks	Ticks

There must have been an original tapeworm of humans living in the gut and passing mature segments in the faeces, as the human carries the final stage of this parasite. When cattle and pigs were domesticated, they became intermediate hosts from eating the mature segments that contained the eggs, so that cysts – containing the immature adult – developed in their muscles. When people eat contaminated meat that has not been cooked sufficiently to kill the cyst contents, the cell wall is digested to release the nascent adult, to begin a new tapeworm.

The adult worms normally cause little pathology, people only knowing they have a worm when they find a mature segment in the faeces, looking rather like a piece of white tape. A more serious problem can, however, occur with the pork tapeworm if the eggs are swallowed directly, e.g. from sewage-contaminated water or a gastric disturbance that causes regurgitation of the mature segment. (This can unfortunately also occur with treatment, so the species of tapeworm must be identified before any treatment is administered.) The immature forms liberated from the eggs then invade the body directly – as they would have done in a pig – and, if they form cysts in the brain, eye or other vital structures, can cause serious problems. This suggests that the pork tapeworm is a more recent parasite than the beef tapeworm in which the life cycle is well established, and causes few problems to the host.

There are other tapeworms of humans that use fish as intermediate hosts, with sometimes extra intermediate organisms such as copepods, leading to complex life cycles. One can only speculate that the original tapeworm – as the final stage is in humans – inhabited our intestines possibly when we emerged from Africa, and that it subsequently developed into different forms that found alternative intermediate hosts by a long sequence of trial and error.

Anthrax

One of the oldest and most feared diseases of cattle is anthrax. It was given this name – the Greek word for coal – by Hippocrates, the father of medicine, because of the blackness of the skin lesion it causes. The disease is also mentioned in the Bible, and the Greek writer Homer was the first to give an account of its devastating effects.

The Roman physician Galen described the disease as well, while anthrax is mentioned in the writings of Virgil too. Outbreaks of anthrax occurred in the medieval period, and in the 18th and 19th centuries there were huge epidemics in the southern part of Europe, killing large numbers of humans as well as domestic animals. These were 'plagues' feared as much as the Black Death because of the rapidity of the illness and its considerable similarity to the pneumonic form of plague. A well person could be dead within 2–3 days.

The causative organism, *Bacillus anthracis*, is a rod-shaped bacterium occurring in pairs and chains, which is comparatively easy to stain, the appearance alone often being sufficient to confirm the diagnosis. As such, it became significant in the history of medicine, as Casimir-Joseph Davine (a French biologist) was the first to identify the anthrax bacillus as a specific microorganism (in 1863), although credit is given to the German Robert Koch, who did not describe it until later.

It is particularly sensitive to oxygen, so if it is exposed to the air it develops spores, which are one of the most resistant forms of life known. They have survived 160°C for an hour and also −78°C, despite thawing and refreezing, while in pastures they have been found viable after 12 years and possibly for as long as 60 years.

Anthrax is predominantly a disease of cattle, so human infection normally starts with cattle handlers or those associated with cattle. The organism enters through a scratch or abrasion on the skin that is in contact with an infected animal, the first sign being a small papule. By the second day, a ring of vesicles surrounds the lesion, which are at first clear but later become bloodstained. The central papule then ulcerates to form the deep, black eschar that gives the disease its name.

Swelling around the lesion can be excessive, causing difficulty in breathing if on the neck, and the person feels unwell. The temperature is not raised except in a serious case, when it indicates that death is not far away. This normally results from inhaling large doses of spores, when the eminently fatal and epidemic pulmonary form of the disease occurs.

Anthrax is still a problem in developing countries and outbreaks among pastoralists continue to occur. Due to the resistant nature of the spores they can remain in the environment for very long periods of time, and where an anthrax-infected animal dies, this becomes contaminated pasture. It might be many years until the wandering cattle return to an infected area, where the anthrax spores are either ingested or inoculated, such as by thistle scratches around the legs or mouth. The spores germinate into the vegetative form, which rapidly invades, the bacteria producing a lethal factor. This directly affects the heart, resulting in the sudden death of the animal. This can be very dramatic, with one moment the animal appearing to be in good health, while in the next it has dropped down dead on the ground. After death, the animal is black from blood that looks as if it has turned to tar.

To the owner of the animal this is a big loss and, either unwittingly or on purpose, he butchers the animal and sells the meat. A serious form of anthrax can develop from swallowing the organism, but most people, fortunately, develop cutaneous anthrax, which is relatively easy to treat with antibiotics. What appears to happen is that those who butcher the carcass or handle the meat get a cutaneous infection, and adequate cooking kills the vegetative form (but not the spores).

Due to drought conditions, cattle from the northern part of Tanzania had been driven to the south to find new grazing within the area where I was working. An animal had died and been slaughtered, and as a result 239 people had developed cutaneous anthrax, from which, luckily, all survived following treatment with a long-lasting form of penicillin. This was at an outlying clinic and it was several days before I was notified.

Rushing to the area and fearing the worst, I was amazed by the casual nature of the medical assistant who had the whole situation perfectly under control and knew exactly what to do. Clearly anthrax was a much commoner problem than I had realized and still responded well to antibiotics, even penicillin.

Unfortunately, because of the way the animal had been slaughtered a new area of infected pasture had been created, and although we were fortunate that no serious cases occurred, the next outbreak might not be so mild. The main control method is to vaccinate animals, but in the developing world this is very difficult to achieve owing to the wandering nature of the herds. If the dead animal is not butchered, the temperature within the carcase will increase sufficiently to kill the vegetative form, but if opened and exposed to the air, resistant spores will form. Hide and bone are also infectious so should be deep buried with lime or incinerated. As dried cow dung makes a good fuel, this can be used to burn the dead animal. Sadly, anthrax-contaminated areas do develop, and although it might be many years before animals return to the same place, the chance of a fresh outbreak is likely.

Louis Pasteur developed the anthrax vaccine in 1881 – the first vaccine to be made from live organisms of the target disease (a live attenuated vaccine). There was initial scepticism, so Pasteur carried out a public trial to demonstrate its effectiveness. He had 50 sheep, two goats and several cows that he divided into two groups; to one he administered the vaccine, and the other remained as controls. Some 30 days later, he gave all the animals anthrax culture by injection, with the result that all the controls died and all of those that had been vaccinated survived.

Once anthrax is recognized, all animals should be vaccinated, while people working with animals or hides might also be offered vaccination. Surprisingly, people who handle contaminated hides are rarely infected, but protective clothing should be provided and a ventilation system installed in the building to remove spores. Ideally, all skins and animal products that could be infected should be disinfected with hypochlorite.

Anthrax is one of the organisms that has been used in bioterrorism, in the infamous postal system attack in the USA in 2001. This was probably a more virulent organism (the Ames strain) that had been produced as a possible biological agent for warfare.

Anthrax was first used for this purpose in 1916 by Scandinavian rebels against the Russian army in Finland. The rebels were supplied with the anthrax by the German High Command. A more notorious use was by the Japanese in Manchuria in 1930, when thousands were killed. Fortunately, the rules of war have as far as we know prevented its further use, but while nations experiment with it, the opportunity for anthrax to be used in bioterrorism remains a distinct possibility.

Brucellosis

A more recently described disease of cattle, pigs and goats is brucellosis, caused by *Brucella melitensis*, *B. abortus* and *B. suis*. The disease and the organism were named after David Bruce (1855–1931), a Scottish pathologist who, while in the British army, identified the bacillus from the spleen of a soldier who had died from it. Indeed, Bruce seems to have been one of the most successful discoverers to have organisms named after him, as he also identified the tsetse fly as the vector responsible for transmitting sleeping sickness, and the trypanasome, *Trypanasoma brucei*, as the infecting organism. As well as being knighted and having other honours conferred on him, he rose to the rank of Major General as the director of army medical services.

Originally called Malta fever (hence *B. melitensis* from Melita, the Roman name for the island), it was a particular problem in the British Army while they were stationed there. Its other name is undulant fever, after its most characteristic symptom. The intermittent fever waxes and wanes for many months and the person feels weak and tired. It varies considerably in severity, with in some cases fatal complications, as occurred in the case investigated by Bruce. The diagnosis is difficult and treatment prolonged, so it is best to try to prevent it in the first place.

Transmission is from drinking raw (unpasteurized) milk or consuming dairy products made from untreated milk, so the practice of drinking warm milk 'fresh from the cow' is really not a good idea. Many of the more recent cases have been in the health-food groups that have promoted goat's milk or goat's cheese, as this is generally not pasteurized and the goat is not so well monitored in the dairy industry as the cow.

The disease is a serious problem in animals, causing considerable economic loss. Brucellosis-free herds need to be built up by eliminating infected animals or, if eradication is not the objective, then vaccination can be used. This is probably a better strategy in developing countries where the disease is a considerable problem. In Sudan and Nigeria, 60% of cattle were found to be infected, with other parts of Africa, South and Central America and the cattle-rearing parts of Asia also having a problem.

Reducing the Risk

Of course, there is a lot we can do to prevent many of the diseases that we acquire from close contact with animals: from the food we eat (Chapter 15), the way domestic animals are cared for, and the keeping of pets. Much emotion surrounds animals, to the extreme case where India has passed a law to prevent the killing of dogs, thereby increasing the incidence of rabies. No other country has such a high rate of rabies, the most awful of diseases and a terrible death, but such is the involvement of religion in politics that simple public health measures are thwarted from doing something about it. Fortunately most other countries can remove unwanted stray animals, and by vaccination reduce the incidence of the disease in the rest. However, there are many other diseases that come from close contact with pets, such as toxocariasis and toxoplasmosis, and no matter how developed the society and well controlled their animals, such diseases are an ever-present risk. As the saying goes, 'A dog is for life, not just for Christmas', meaning that it should always be cared for, though from a public health aspect this can also be interpreted that this potential source of infection, polluting the environment with its excrement and passing on parasites, is with us for a very long time. There is no safe pet; every animal has risk attached to it, no matter how well it is cared for.

The implications of looking after pets are something that few people think about. Dogs and cats are both carnivores, so have predominantly meat diets, meaning that their excrement is high in nitrogen, which when deposited on the soil alters the local flora. In areas where people regularly take their dogs for walks outside the designated built-up area – which means that they are not legally obliged to clean up after their animals – can be seen areas of altered vegetation quite alien to that in the rest of the surrounding terrain. This might seem a small matter, but damaging the environment in whatever way it is done is a concern of many people at this time.

This high meat diet, although consisting of scraps, horsemeat and other types of protein, is not only expensive, but would be welcomed as a source of protein in many parts of the world. Pet owners spend more money on feeding their animals than many families do on trying to keep themselves alive in the developing world. One only has to look at the number of shelves devoted to pet food in the local supermarket to realize how much money is spent on dogs and cats.

An article in *This is Money* of 28 September 2011 estimated that, excluding the price of purchasing the pet, it costs in the region of £17,000 for the upkeep of a dog or cat over its lifetime. However, this does not take into account inflation, with the likelihood that this will be in the region of £19,000 by 2026.

Is having a pet such a necessity? By not keeping a pet, not only would disease carried by animals be reduced, but the environment would be better protected and more done for the rest of humanity.

The Animal Connection

12

Animal Origins

In the previous chapter, diseases of animals that affect humans (zoonoses) have been mentioned, but the connection with animals is probably more subtle and long lasting.

Smallpox, measles, mumps, diphtheria, pertussis (whooping cough) and scarlet fever were all originally diseases of animals, as can be seen in their DNA sequences, but evolved into exclusively human infections. This change might have occurred during the agricultural revolution (around 5000 BC), when animals were first domesticated. It was the parasite's adaptability to finding new and more successful hosts that led to the transition.

Initially, the organism would have continued to affect both the animal and the human host, but if the purely human cycle conferred advantages, then this would have been selected as the more successful. This could be by two different mechanisms, either the single organism changed host completely or different strains developed to continue in each host. Such a process is more likely to occur in viral diseases as their construction is more malleable than that of bacteria.

The measles virus is most closely related to the rinderpest virus of cattle and probably originated around 5000 years ago, developing as a separate organism to infect humans, while the rinderpest virus continued as a devastating animal disease. Although rinderpest is a disease of animals, it has probably caused a huge loss of human life as well. So associated are many tribes with cattle that to lose them from disease brings poverty and starvation to their owners. The Kikuyu tribe in Kenya considered the introduction of rinderpest the greatest ill that had befallen their people, while their great enemies the Masai (or Maasai), who are even more dependent on their cattle, were decimated. Towards the end of the 19th century, the Masai were the dominant tribe in East Africa, but by the beginning of the 20th century

© R. Webber 2015. *Disease Selection: The Way Disease Changed the World* (R. Webber)

some 90% of their cattle had been killed by disease and many of them inflicted by smallpox, so reducing them to the minor status they now have.

HIV Infection

The most serious communicable disease of the modern era, that caused by human immunodeficiency virus (HIV), originated from an animal source.

In June 1981, the Centers for Disease Control (CDC, now the Centers for Disease Control and Prevention) in the USA reported five cases of *Pneumocystis jiroveci* (previously called *P. carini*) pneumonia. In the following month, 15 or more cases of this normally rare disease were reported and, in addition, 26 cases of Kaposi's sarcoma, an unusual tumour. The common feature was that all of these cases were in homosexual men. By the end of 1981, acquired immune deficiency syndrome (AIDS), as it was called, was being reported from countries in Europe. In Belgium and France, an AIDS-like illness was noted among people originating from Africa, leading to investigations in Rwanda and Zaire (now the Democratic Republic of the Congo), where many AIDS patients were found. At the same time, an aggressive form of Kaposi's sarcoma was reported from Zambia and a new disease, called 'slim disease', was described in Uganda. These were all found to be manifestations of AIDS. The African disease was transmitted heterosexually, as opposed to how the condition was first found to be spread.

A search was made for the source of the disease of African origin, and several earlier outbreaks, which were self-limiting, discovered. Two strains of the HIV virus were causing infection, the original HIV1 found throughout Africa and other parts of the world, and HIV2, a less serious infection found predominantly in West Africa. A search was then made among animals, and HIV1 was found in chimpanzees and HIV2 in the Sooty Mangabey monkey. Sadly, the monkey and chimpanzee had become favoured items of the diet, particularly in the Cameroon and Congo forest area, and it is thought that this predilection for 'bush meat' had brought humans into sufficiently close contact, and that when animals were butchered, blood contamination took place. Transfusion of blood has been a potent method of infection, so contamination of a wound with chimpanzee or monkey blood could quite easily have done the same.

The chimpanzee does not appear to be ill, although it contains large amounts of virus in its blood, so it seems to be the natural reservoir of infection. Genetic analysis suggests that HIV originated sometime around 1908 within the chimpanzee, while the first recorded human epidemic was in 1959, near Kinshasa. In the 1970s, it entered the commercial sex industry, and at a later date the homosexual community, as described above.

It was probably the change in sex habits, especially in the number of partners, that led to the selection of more virulent strains, allowing greater spread. It did not matter to the virus that people were dying, as owing to the large number of sexual contacts the disease was easily transmitted. It might never have taken off and become a global pandemic if it had not been for this sexual liberation. However, by the same reasoning, if proper preventive methods are used, it can be anticipated that strains of lesser virulence will be selected for, as is already showing signs of happening (see Chapter 3). This will depend upon strict adherence to methods of prevention, especially while under treatment.

When I was first working in Tanzania we had no cases of HIV infection and I can remember reading about the unusual infection in homosexual men that had been reported by the CDC. It was not long before we discovered our first case and within a short period of time, not only was it a pan-African problem, but a global one as well. It was horrifying to see the speed at which it was travelling and how quickly it found its way into new areas. There are now estimated to be 35 million people with HIV in the world, 19 million of them being infected but not knowing that they are.

HIV has become a serious problem because of the damage it causes to the immune system. Individuals lose their normal defence mechanisms, opening them up to a number of infections that they would not normally be susceptible to, such as unexplained chronic diarrhoea, recurrent pneumonia and candida (fungal) infection of the mouth and throat. There has been an increase in more established infections as well, particularly tuberculosis (TB), malaria, leishmaniasis and intractable scabies. The TB problem is particularly serious, with an extra 0.52 million deaths from TB in HIV-positive persons in 2008.

HIV is poorly transmitted, with only about 5% becoming infected after exposure by the sexual route. But the more sexual contacts, the greater the risk of contracting infection, and such factors as other sexually transmitted infections (STIs) also determine the likelihood of getting the disease.

The initial fear of the disease has been lessened by the development of drugs and the good response made by most people to treatment. However the disease is still not curable, and if the drugs are not taken continuously then serious complications develop. There can be no complacency that HIV is no longer a problem or that it is just a matter of time before a vaccine is developed. Attempts have been made ever since the virus was isolated, including some high-profile demonstrations by scientists trying out vaccines on themselves, but all to no avail. The problem is that the virus changes its antigenic form so rapidly that the body has no time to develop immunity against it. What is particularly worrying is the development of an AIDS superbug that threatens treatment regimes. If this was to become widely disseminated, then present treatment regimes would be largely ineffective. Prevention is still better than cure.

As a species, humans have been through a long association with disease-causing organisms and some of our earlier familiarity with them can sometimes be of value. Such might be the discovery of the mutated gene

CCR5-Δ32, which protects some 1–5% of Europeans from HIV infection, and probably helped segments of the population survive the plague epidemics. It is curious that previous experience of one disease should have produced individuals that are protected from another that had not even come into existence.

Severe Acute Respiratory Syndrome

One of the most successful viral adaptations has been that of influenza, which was described on Chapter 10. Not only is it a disease of birds and pigs, but new variants can develop that become exclusively human infections. No other disease process is so efficient at mixing genetic material from animals and humans to produce new strains of disease.

This mixing of human and animal genetic material in the development of new influenza strains is most profound in the southern part of China, where animals are kept alive ready to be eaten, in the most unhygienic conditions. This seems to have been the manner in which one of the most serious new diseases, severe acute respiratory syndrome (SARS), originated.

In February 2003, a businessman who had been travelling in China was admitted to a hospital in Hanoi, Vietnam, suffering from fever, cough and difficulty in breathing. His condition worsened so he requested to be transferred to Hong Kong, where, despite intensive care, he died. In the hospital in Hanoi several healthcare workers contracted a similar disease, and the attending doctor and a nurse died. A search was made for the organism responsible, which was at first thought to be an emergent strain of influenza, but subsequently a new coronavirus was identified.

Tracing the original case back, it was discovered that there had been a number of cases of a severe pneumonia in Guangdong Province (Canton), southern China, in which 1 in 30 people had died. The attending specialist travelled to Hong Kong for a wedding where, in the early stages of the infection himself, he infected all the people in a lift in the hotel where he was staying. One of these was the case that came to Hanoi, another a person from Singapore and the third a lady returning to her home in Toronto, Canada. Each of these cases then became centres of epidemics, which demanded strict quarantine measures to contain them. After draconian measures, especially in China, the last case recovered at the end of July 2003. By that time, there had been 8422 cases and 916 deaths.

While major efforts were being made to contain the human epidemics, a search was made among the first cases discovered in Guangdong for a possible cause. Several of these were food handlers and 66 of them had antibodies to the SARS virus. The search then shifted to the animals they were looking after and antibodies were found in racoon dogs, ferret badgers, cynomolgus macaques, fruit bats, snakes, wild pigs and masked palm civets. The highest level of antibodies was found in the masked palm civet, which was thought to be the main source, but may not be the definitive reservoir.

Fortunately, there have been no further cases of SARS, but the danger of exotic food sources (and the related poor conditions in which some animals are kept alive for the table) is highlighted. Hopefully, measures have and will continue to be taken to prevent such potentially lethal epidemics from happening again.

Creutzfeldt–Jakob Disease

While we may express our amazement at the eating habits of southern China, the next epidemic of an animal-related disease was to occur much closer to home. The first sign of a new disease appeared in cattle in England in 1986. This was called bovine spongiform encephalopathy (BSE) or, more commonly, mad-cow disease, after the disorientated manner of the affected animal, which staggered around in an uncoordinated fashion, frequently falling over. The new disease had all the appearances of scrapie, a disease previously restricted to sheep.

It did not take long to discover that cattle had indeed been fed the remains of sheep, with the possibility that some of the feed contained scrapie-infected remains. It seems almost inconceivable that the agricultural feed industry should incorporate animal parts in a food that is to be given to herbivores, but such was the desire for profit over the possible health implications that this is indeed what was done. Scrapie had been transmitted to cattle, and if this had happened with sheep-to-cattle then might it not also happen with cattle-to-humans?

Sure enough, the first cases of a new debilitating disease that had a similar clinical presentation to a rare human condition called Creutzfeldt–Jakob disease (CJD), appeared in 1995. This was linked to the eating of beef, and the mince used in the making of beefburgers can come from many different animals, one or more of which may have had BSE. As the incubation period of CJD was 4–5 years, and the new disease and CJD were very similar, this was likely to be the period of time during which people had been eating potentially infected meat. This also meant that the number of cases of what came to be called new-variant CJD (vCJD) could have been enormous.

By the end of 1995 three cases were confirmed, one of which died, after which there was a gradual increase up to the year 2000, when 28 cases were diagnosed. This appeared to be the peak of the epidemic because there was then a steady decline, with one fatal case in 2008, three in 2009 and three in 2010. Four more cases were diagnosed after this, making 174 cases altogether. In addition, there were six cases in France and one each in Ireland, Italy, Canada and the USA, with three of the French cases and those in Canada and the USA considered to have contracted their infection in the UK. It certainly could have been a lot worse, but to die from vCJD was a slow, lingering, awful death, in a disease that could have been completely avoided in the first place.

Bats

As well as contracting diseases from animals, as described above, animals can also be reservoirs of disease. The multimammate rat in Lassa fever or the monkey in yellow fever are called reservoirs because they act as sources of infection for these diseases, but do not noticeably suffer from illness themselves. Many animals are reservoirs of disease, with the rat and the dog perhaps the most important, but increased interest has been taken in the bat as a likely new source of infection.

The vampire bat was first discovered to be a reservoir of rabies during work in Trinidad in the 1930s. Subsequently, it was discovered that insectivorous and frugivorous bats could also carry the rabies virus, as demonstrated when two explorers went into a cave in West Africa and contracted the fatal disease. Then, in 1999, a new viral infection appeared in pig farmers in Malaysia that presented as an encephalitis, with a high case-fatality rate of 40–70%, and subsequently called Nipah. Fruit-eating bats of the genus *Pteropus* (flying foxes) were found to be reservoirs of the disease, and wherever this bat was found, including India, Bangladesh, Thailand, Malaysia, Indonesia, Cambodia, China, Papua New Guinea and Australia, the Nipah virus was present.

The same genus of bats and the virus are found in Madagascar, but so far there have been no outbreaks of disease. Another bat genus, *Eidon*, which belongs to the same family of bats and is widely distributed in Africa, also tested positive for antibodies to the virus.

In the outbreak of Nipah in Bangladesh, pigs became infected from eating fruit contaminated with the saliva or urine of bats. Transmission from one pig to another, and to humans, was mainly by droplet infection, but the tissues of pigs are also infected, so handling them, especially at their slaughter, could lead to infection. Horses, goats, sheep, cats and dogs can also be infected with Nipah.

Another viral infection related to Nipah and also to the same kind of bat, but so far restricted to Australia, is Hendra. This is a disease predominantly of horses in which it has caused serious economic loss, although there have been only a few human cases. Infected pasture is contaminated with bat fetal tissue and fluid during delivery, and is subsequently grazed by horses.

Ebola, like Lassa, is a highly infectious haemorrhagic fever, for which a reservoir of infection is being sought, with the bat the most likely candidate. Fruit bats have been found to carry the virus and infection may occur from direct contact with bats or their excreta, as well as from infected humans. Several caves in sub-Saharan Africa have been found to be inhabited by bats carrying the virus, so should be avoided. Also, like Lassa, infection in childhood might produce some immunity, but this has not been established yet. It is thought that the recent large outbreak of Ebola that caused so many deaths in Guinea, Sierra Leone and Liberia started from children catching bats that they then cooked and ate.

Cross-species Transmission

The animals that we have domesticated or come into contact with have had a longer evolutionary history than humans, and so more opportunity to acquire diseases. At the same time, parasites exploited new ways to extend their range and in so doing found ways of moving across the species divide to affect humans. We have made this easier for them by hunting and killing animals or keeping them in unhygienic conditions. Even our domestic animals and pets, which are looked after with care, just by their association with humans provide opportunities for transmission. Natural selection may have helped us reach the level of sophistication that we now live in, but we have also facilitated diseases to work against us.

Not Clean

13

Neonatal Tetanus

The beautiful but remote island of St Kilda, off the West Coast of Scotland, was occupied for at least 1000 years by a very resilient group of islanders who mainly lived on seabirds, fish and the few vegetables they could cultivate on the limited area of arable land available. They were a small but self-sufficient community, passing on their skills from generation to generation and very successfully maintaining a way of life that had seen them survive terrible storms, shortages of food, lack of contact and deprivation. But on Wednesday 27 August 1930, this all came to an end; they asked to be removed and resettled on the mainland.

It was not any single event that had caused this decision, but the community had gradually declined in size and they now felt it was no longer viable. There were not sufficient young people to continue the community and soon there would not be enough to look after the increasingly older generation. This, however, was not because the younger people had left to find work on the mainland, the fate of many an island community, but because there had been a run of infant deaths and there were now not enough surviving children.

The community had been well provided for with a resident nurse and minister, who had both tried to understand why infants were dying. The cause was all too obvious, the terrible shaking and paralysis of neonatal tetanus, but why should it be so serious here and carry away the generation that was to keep the community going? The nurse and the minister did have a theory about why this was happening, but try as they could to persuade the people, traditional practice could not be changed and, sadly, the infants kept on dying.

The main seabird the people caught was the fulmar, taking the young from the cliffs and cooking them to extract the oil. This was a precious commodity, used for many purposes, but one they considered essential was to treat the umbilical stump of the newborn infant. The fulmar oil might stand on the shelf for many months and there was no way in which it could be kept sterile, and some 5–10 days after it had been placed on the umbilicus, the newborn would have difficulty in sucking. Soon after that there would be rigidity of the muscles, followed by generalized convulsions, and the infant would soon die.

It just seemed impossible to convince the mothers not to use the fulmar oil; this was how it had always been done and there was no reason why they should change things now. However, this was the reason the infants were dying: the oil was contaminated with tetanus bacilli, and 1000 years of history came to an end because of this traditional practice.

Local methods of treating the umbilical stump after the cord has been cut are practised in many parts of the world and, unfortunately, the story of what happened in St Kilda is all too frequently heard. One of the favourite poultices used in developing countries is cow dung. This is already loaded with tetanus bacilli so is an almost certain way of infecting the newborn infant, but it is a very hard practice to stop. Once the child reaches 6–8 weeks of age it can receive its first dose of triple vaccine, but many an infant still dies before it is allowed to live this long.

Trachoma

The most important cause of blindness, trachoma, is widespread in the drier parts of the world, with an estimated 360 million cases in 1985. This had been reduced to 41 million by 2009 using the simplest of control measures – washing the face with water. Initially, mass treatments using antibiotic eye ointment were conducted, but getting people to wash their faces at regular intervals has been a far more sustainable method.

The main sign of trachoma is 'red eye', and the discharge that is produced is transferred by fingers, families and flies. The common scenario is the large family, living in squalid conditions in which the mother uses a cloth or her fingers to wipe the secretions from the eyes of one child, and the same cloth is subsequently used on another child. All the time, annoying little flies (*Musca sorbens*) are attracted by the same secretions and help in their spread.

Flies breed in animal and human excreta, so the removal of these and the use of proper latrines are methods of control. This, with the provision of water supplies, can do much to reduce the diseases of poor hygiene. It might seem surprising that the best method of preventing people from going blind is to give them a water supply!

Yaws and Syphilis

A group of disfiguring diseases that were at one time common in the world and known as the endemic treponematoses (named after the causative organism) have largely been controlled by mass treatment and improvements in hygiene. The commonest of these was yaws, which in its tertiary stage led to gross damage of the skin and bone, leading to hideous deformities. Campaigns of mass treatment in the last century that used a single injection of penicillin G reduced the distribution of yaws to a few parts of West Africa, Congo, Papua New Guinea, Indonesia and Timor-Leste, where it is still found.

The evolution of this group of diseases appears to have taken place in comparatively recent times. Yaws, pinta and endemic syphilis are all transmitted by *Treponema* spp., with the organism causing endemic syphilis identical to the *T. pallidum* of venereal syphilis. Serological tests for syphilis are positive in the endemic disease, and the appearance under the microscope of samples of *T. pallidum* isolated from cases of the two diseases is exactly the same, yet the illnesses are quite different. In endemic syphilis, the primary lesion of a raised mucous plaque is commonly found at the angle of the mouth, after which a florid skin infection develops. Moist papules under the arms and between the buttocks and a maculopapular rash on the trunk and limbs are the only signs that resemble the venereal disease. There is never the primary chancre associated with sexual contact, nor the nervous and cardiovascular complications of the tertiary disease.

Endemic syphilis is now only found in localized areas of the Sahel region of Africa and in Saudi Arabia and Yemen, where it is known as Bejel or Njovera, and is becoming increasingly rare. If you have had endemic syphilis then you are protected from the more serious disease of venereal syphilis, so there are no major efforts to eliminate it. Like trachoma, endemic syphilis is found in situations of poor hygiene, where people crowd together and contact with lesions and their secretions can readily occur.

There has been much speculation about where syphilis came from. The first clear epidemic appeared in the army of Charles VIII when he attacked Naples in 1494. This has been traced back to mercenaries joining his army who had served with Columbus on his transatlantic voyage. There is even an account of Columbus having had sexual relations with the local inhabitants, so it would seem almost certain that members of his crew had done likewise.

These findings indicate an origin for syphilis in the Americas, which is further supported by characteristic changes in the bones and teeth of pre-Columbian skeletons. There did not seem to be changes in skeletons on the European side of the Atlantic, except for some signs suggestive of syphilis found on skeletons of monks from an English monastery. These were dated between 1300 and 1450, well before Columbus's voyage, but controversy surrounds this isolated finding. It still seems unlikely, though, that venereal syphilis should have a New World origin when endemic syphilis almost certainly originated in Africa.

With the identical nature of *T. pallidum* in both endemic and venereal syphilis, this link between the two diseases goes without question, so why should the organism, having found a highly successful way of spreading itself by the sexual route, revert to the less effective method used by endemic syphilis? The transition may have taken place between the non-venereal and venereal forms of the disease in the Americas, as one of the treponematoses, pinta, is found in the tropical areas of Central and South America, but this does not rule out an Old World origin for the *Treponema* spirochaete. It would seem more likely that the non-venereal form accompanied the small groups of travellers, originally from Africa, who crossed the land bridge between Asia and the Americas and, somewhere along the route, the more effective sexual method of transmission evolved. So *T. pallidum* may still have originated in Africa in endemic syphilis, but became a sexually transmitted disease only when it reached the Americas. Perhaps further clues will come from skeletons in Siberia or the sequencing of the genetic make-up of *T. pallidum*.

Handwashing

We are all taught by our mothers to wash our hands after going to the toilet or before meals, but it is surprising how important this advice really is. When the number of diseases that can be prevented by the simple expedient of washing the hands with soap and water is counted up, it comes to the remarkable figure of 102, and this might not be all of them. Personal hygiene is a life-saving practice and its promotion in the developing world by the provision of water supplies is probably the most cost-effective health strategy that can be provided. This is the simplest and most valuable public health method that we can undertake.

There is no need to use antiseptic solutions, in fact they might even potentiate some infections; as mentioned below, soap and water are perfectly effective. Also there is no advantage to using liquid soap over solid soap; like so many things this has been an advertising triumph for the detergent industry – to get people to use more expensive liquid soap. It has no advantages over the solid tablets of soap we used to be more familiar with. Indeed, the action of rubbing the solid soap between the hands has a mechanical effect and helps to get the soap into all the recesses of our hands. Ordinary soap and water can do more for us than many of the treatments and expensive remedies that have been produced to take their place.

It is surprising that our common method of greeting each other, the handshake, appears to be designed to transmit infection from one person to another. Although you might have washed your hands, you cannot be sure that the other person has, and what is even more contaminating is that greeting is often associated with eating, that people shake hands just before they are about to sit down for a meal.

The shaking of hands is depicted on Greek statues as far back as the 5th century BC and was thought to indicate that no weapon was held in the hand, similar to the wave of the hand from further away. However such indicators are not now required, and with several parasitic diseases or epidemics of influenza, a more deadly weapon is transmitted by the handshake.

The traditional Indian style of greeting practised in much of Asia – that of placing both hands together without touching the other person – is not only more hygienic but probably has more ancient origins. I was also impressed by the Nubian style of greeting still practised in the northern part of Sudan, where two people meeting each other place their right hand on the other person's shoulder. This is depicted in carvings in the Temple of Amun, in Naqa, a ruined city just north of Khartoum and dating from the first century AD, but it might have been an even older Egyptian form of greeting. There are many ways in which we could greet the other person without using the most potent one for transferring infection.

Education

Much of ill health is due to ignorance or traditional practice, allowing disease to select against us. Traditions take a long time to change and it is only after concerted effort and education that change may be effective. This is a difficult problem in developing countries, but even in the more developed countries it can be equally hard, with smoking being a good example. One only has to look at films made in the 1950s or before to see how entrenched and accepted this was in society. It was in the same decade that the pioneering work by Doll and Hill was carried out showing the link between smoking and lung cancer, yet it has taken until recently for a reversal of attitudes. Change comes slowly and education is as valuable a method to combat disease as all the medical methods that have so far been devised.

Too Clean

14

Poliomyelitis

Poliomyelitis is a disease of poor sanitation, surviving in conditions of poverty in many parts of the world. Young children meet the virus and develop immunity, with only a few going on to have the paralytic disease. However, once the state of sanitation is improved there is not this constant exposure at a young age and, sadly, the rewards for improving the hygiene of the community are the chance of getting polio at an older age, when the incidence of paralytic disease is increased.

This was what happened to perhaps the greatest president there has ever been of the USA, Franklin D. Roosevelt (Fig. 14.1). He contracted polio in 1921 at the age of 39 when he was campaigning for the presidency of James Cox, with himself as vice president. Fortunately, he survived the worst kind of paralysis and went on to complete three terms of office and win the presidency four times, the only person ever to achieve this. It was the greatly improved state of health in the community that had kept him free of infection when he was young, but the polio virus was still circulating and, tragically, he became infected in later life.

Brought up in a well-to-do family, Roosevelt would never have been exposed to the polio virus as a child and therefore been able to develop immunity. When he was canvassing, it is likely that he visited disadvantaged areas where the polio virus was circulating, and so developed the more serious form of the disease as an adult. He suffered severely, and initially was almost completely paralysed. Gradually, he regained the use of all of his musculature, except for his legs. During this time his wife Eleanor – niece of President Theodore Roosevelt – not only encouraged and supported him, but became his eyes and ears at all the meetings.

He never walked again and spent the rest of his life in a wheelchair. He was, however, a big man and when the going in a meeting became tough, he would haul himself up to his full height, which often had a dramatic effect on the opposition.

© R. Webber 2015. *Disease Selection: The Way Disease Changed the World* (R. Webber)

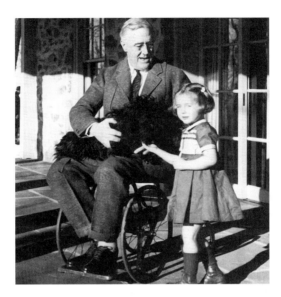

Fig. 14.1. Franklin D. Roosevelt, who contracted polio when he was 39. (*Images of American Political History*, 1941, public domain.)

His mother had tried to persuade him to retire – a voice of common sense against a spirit of determination – it was certainly a close shave with disease that we got such a superb president.

Would Roosevelt have been such a good president if he had not had to go through the battle with polio which brought out such determination in him? We will never know.

One never wishes for anyone to have to go through such a difficult period and live with a disability, but it often does bring out the best in people. In more recent times, there has been growing admiration for the sporting success achieved in the Paralympic Games, which allows disabled people to compete against each other in the same way as the Olympic Games. Most of these disablements are now due to amputations resulting from accidents or war, but if the games had been held several decades ago, the participants would probably have been mainly polio disabled.

On one of my medical rounds in Solomon Islands I arrived at a village in the morning to witness what looked like half a man make his way down to the beach. He had contracted polio and both his lower limbs were so withered away that it almost seemed he had no legs at all. In compensation, he had huge shoulders and arm muscles with which he propelled himself to the water's edge and, once in the sea, swam with considerable power. Reaching his canoe he would easily lift himself in, fitting in the bottom more easily than if he had his original legs. Once he started paddling, it was as though he had a motor driving the canoe, such was the strength of his arms and the reduced weight of his withered legs.

He would happily fish all day, as was the traditional occupation of most of the men of this village, but he was always the champion, bringing in more fish than anybody else – he had turned his disability into an advantage.

Allergic Conditions

There has been a noticeable increase in the allergic diseases of asthma, hay fever and ulcerative colitis, and one of the theories for this is that we have become too clean. As children during the war years we would be outside all the time, playing with what we found and coming home thoroughly dirty, to be chastised by our mothers but never prevented from doing what seemed to be natural for children at that time. Since then, attitudes have changed; spurred on by the advertising industry to sterilize and to be clean, mothers have prevented their children from getting dirty. We are surrounded by microbes of all kinds, and coming into contact with many of them during childhood builds up our immune history, so if we are prevented from this experience, we will not have the opportunity to acquire this immunity or the capacity to deal with meeting these organisms later on in life.

In support of this theory, Western people have been found to have less diversity of bacteria in their guts than hunter–gatherers, who are noticeably free of allergies. Also, people with allergies have less diversity of bacteria than people without allergies. A life outdoors has been found to increase our diversity of bacteria.

When we are born, lactobacilli in our mother's vagina coat us at birth and inhabit our gut as our first bacteria. They are increased by breastfeeding, protecting the newborn from microbes that might harm them. However, if the child is delivered by caesarean section this does not happen, and if it is not breastfed it is at an even greater disadvantage. After its initial protection, the infant is exposed to a wide range of organisms, to which it mounts an immune response. Later on in life, if any bacteria have not been met with before, the immune system appears to overreact and produce an allergic response.

During this vital stage in childhood, when immunity is being built up, a course of antibiotics will reduce the bacterial flora and the opportunity to develop immunity to it. The greater the number of courses of antibiotics in early life, the greater is the likelihood of developing allergies. Of the different types of bacteria, actinobacteria are more common in allergic individuals and bifidobacteria predominate in non-allergic individuals.

More specifically, Martin Blaser and his research team based at New York University have been interested in *Helicobacter pylori*. This lives in the lining of the stomach, the only type of bacterium found there because of the lethal nature of stomach acidity. It has somehow evolved to survive in this unusual place, producing a mild inflammation of the stomach wall. This was previously thought to be harmful and a precursor to stomach ulcers and cancer, but it now seems that it has a regulatory effect on immunity, preventing it from overreacting, as occurs in an allergic response. By administering antibiotics, particularly at a young age, *H. pylori* is killed off and its protective effect destroyed. There may also be a relationship between antibiotic administration and childhood obesity, as mentioned in Chapter 15.

Clostridium difficile, which produces a chronic debilitating diarrhoea, used to be a rare infection, but has increased at the expense of other gut bacteria killed off by the overuse of antibiotics. The situation has been made worse by the use of alcohol hand gels, promoted on cruise liners to reduce Noro virus outbreaks, and now also promoted in the home; these are not effective against *C. difficile* spores, and so give a false sense of protection. Soap has been a valuable method of washing the hands for a considerable period of time and still remains the best substance for this purpose in the majority of situations. Once again, the advertising industry has done us a disservice by using the banner of cleanliness.

Another value of gut bacteria, particularly *Lactobacillus* and *Bifidobacteria*, may be in controlling our mood, dampening down anxiety and preventing mood swings. This is still a controversial area of research, but it might show that replacing gut bacteria by probiotics, after their elimination by antibiotics, particularly in the young and the old, might not only restore our gut flora but improve our mood as well.

As well as bacteria, the larger parasitic worms have been found to dampen down our immune system. Hookworms and roundworms are able to live in our intestines because of the substances they secrete, which inhibit attempts by the body to eliminate them. Infestation by parasitic worms is more common in developing countries, where allergic conditions are rare and it seems that a few worms do you more good than harm. Attempts are being made to isolate the substance produced by intestinal parasitic worms that protect the gut from overreacting, while some people have successfully treated their ulcerative colitis by purposely infecting themselves with a small dose of hookworms.

There may be a connection between these two theories, because parasitic worms will have their complement of bacteria as well, and as they live within the human intestines they are likely to be colonized by the same bacteria that we have. If certain types of bacteria bring benefit to us, then it is perfectly possible that they will do the same for nematodes, which have their own set of intestines. Antibiotic use will destroy these friendly bacteria within the worm just as they will within our gut, possibly causing problems for the parasite as well as for us.

Immune Stimulation

We are compromising ourselves and the generations of evolutionary steps it has taken humans to build up their immune systems to protect them against disease. We are preventing immune mechanisms from coming into contact with the necessary bacterial stimuli in our overzealous attempts to become too clean.

The Food We Eat

15

Dietary Fibre

There used to be a medical condition called essential hypertension, in which blood pressure increased with age so that in later life you were more susceptible to strokes and other fatal conditions. Hugh Trowell (1904–1989), working in Mulago Hospital, Kampala, Uganda, attached to Makerere Medical School, routinely took the blood pressure of the many patients he saw during the course of his medical practice. To his surprise, he did not find the same rise of blood pressure with age in the African population that came to his clinic. There seemed to be a different situation in the population in East Africa where he was working. Was this a racial or a genetic difference, or was there another cause?

Trowell, with his interest in nutrition, suspected it was something to do with diet. After some searching, he noticed that Africans consumed considerably less salt than Europeans and hypothesized that this might be the reason. Salt was difficult to come by in this part of the world, the main source being certain grasses that produced a salty taste when burnt. Large studies have since been undertaken that support his theory and, as a result, the advice given now is that salt intake should be limited.

Hugh Trowell was a wonderful character and I remember a lecture he gave in which he showed a series of pictures of faecal deposits. He had gone round his African neighbourhood where people used to go to defecate and recorded his findings, not to demonstrate the poor state of hygiene of the area, which the exercise certainly could have done, but to record the nature of the faecal pile. The obvious finding was the large volume of stool compared with the small, solid contribution of the average Western person. He coined the term 'dietary fibre' to illustrate that the average African consumed large quantities of fruit and vegetables, the remains of which were excreted in the stool, producing bulk and speeding up transit time. Similar to his observations on hypertension, Trowell had noticed that the common Western diseases, coronary heart disease, diabetes and bowel cancer, were virtually unknown in his African population, and he suspected that this was due to dietary differences, as demonstrated by the faecal output. As a result of this pioneering work, we are now recommended to eat our 'Five a Day'.

The considerable contribution made by Hugh Trowell has never been acknowledged and his name is hardly known today. As well as his work on the aetiology of Western diseases, he also described kwashiorkor as a separate disease from marasmus and introduced Denis Burkitt to the childhood tumour that would later be called Burkitt's lymphoma (see Chapter 16).

Balanced Diet

Most people think of the human body as a kind of machine, rather like a motor car; as long as you keep on putting fuel (food) into it, it will keep going. Nothing, however, could be further from the truth – we are what we eat, as one of the popular slogans describes the process. The human body is made up of numerous different kinds of cells, which are born, mature and die, to be replaced by new cells. These are all made from the nutrients we consume, so in effect what we eat becomes our body. Apart from brain cells, it is estimated that we replace our entire body (including our skeleton) about every 20 years. So if we exist on junk food we can expect a junk result; it really is 'rubbish in, rubbish out'.

There are four main kinds of foods – proteins, fats, carbohydrates and sugars – as well as vitamins and essential minerals, all of which we need in differing quantities at different times in our lives. When we are growing up we need more proteins to provide for an expanding body frame, but once this has been achieved, at about the age of 18 years, we no longer need a high protein diet, yet the average adult consumes far more protein than they require. Similarly, with the energy foods – fats, carbohydrates and sugars – if we lead a sedentary life then the quantity required is less than when following active pursuits.

Insulin controls the nutrient levels of the body and if too much food is consumed then it is stored as fat. Fats in food are high-energy constituents, but if they are not utilized there is little conversion required to store them in fat cells in the body, so it is normally better to try to cut down on fat consumption. When required, fat is broken down into sugars, but the reverse also happens, so if excess sugars are consumed they are converted into fat. Protein is also converted into fat if it is not required in body growth or repair, and much of the obesity problem is caused by eating beef protein.

There is good evidence that a high-protein diet is more satiating – satisfying the appetite – and it has been used, mainly in celebrity circles, as a form of dieting. However, cattle fed on grain (which supply the main type of beef found in supermarkets) rather than natural pasture have in-creased fat content, so the result is excess fat in the diet.

Infant Feeds and Breast Milk

Like all cells in the body, fat cells develop in the infant and if it is overfed then the number of fat cells increases. A fat cell can lose its fat content in later life but it still remains as an additional cell so there is always a ten-dency for it to be filled again. Fat babies, therefore, tend to become fat adults and the proper feeding of infants can do much to reduce childhood, and later adult, obesity.

Human breast milk is for human babies, whereas cow's milk is for baby cows, and they are not the same. Cow's milk contains a higher butter fat content, so artificial infant food manufacturers have to manipulate this difference in trying to produce an equivalent formula. Generally, they err on the side of a higher fat content and make this appear to be the ideal, with a picture of a fat baby on the outside of the container. Always the best strategy is to breastfeed the child for as long as the mother is able and, if possible, continue into the weaning period, going straight on to solid foods, rather than using artificial infant formulas at all.

As mentioned in the previous chapter, the infant is covered in lacto-bacilli when it is born, and breast milk contains an additional source of these bacteria, as well as other valuable constituents that artificial milk formula does not have. After this initial protection, the infant acquires a bacterial flora similar to that of its mother. Not only are these bacteria useful in inhabiting the gut, where they aid in digestion, but they also protect the infant from disease-producing bacteria. The destruction of these bacteria by the use of antibiotics, as mentioned in Chapter 14, can have adverse effects. This is more serious in the child under 3 years of age, and antibiotics should not be given to children of this age if at all possible.

As is mentioned below, the agricultural industry has found that giving low-dose antibiotics to animals promotes their growth in body fat, and it can be hypothesized that a similar increase in fat content could happen in humans. Analysis of the Avon Longitudinal Study of Parents and Children (ALSPAC) began in 1991 and, as one of its associated results, found that children given antibiotics in the first 6 months of life did indeed become fatter. Although this is not the continuous low dose of antibiotics as ad-ministered to farm animals, an ordinary course of antibiotics given early in life has a similar effect.

Sadly, this is all too common, with antibiotics being administered for a whole range of childhood conditions for which they are probably not required. Not only is this leading to an increase in allergic conditions (Chapter 14) but to childhood obesity as well.

Cow's Milk

There is considerable myth surrounding the drinking of cow's milk, in that it is healthy and good for us. It is good for the growing child as it contains fat and protein, but in the adult this is not required; indeed, the additional fat is likely to be added to the excess that furs up the arteries. Milk and dairy products are a source of calcium, but there are many other sources, including water from chalk and limestone areas.

The dairy industry has a continuing dilemma on its hands, as milk is only produced by pregnant cows, and pregnant cows produce baby calves. Half of these on average will be males so will not grow up to become more milk producers, and need to be slaughtered at an appropriate age to be turned into beef. The more beef that is produced, the more milk there will be also, so the dairy industry has tried to avoid an excess by encouraging us to drink more milk. Similarly, at times when milk (including cheeses and other milk products) is sufficient, then the advertising is reversed and we are told that eating more beef (mostly grain fed) will turn us into muscular men wearing kilts. Neither of these exhortations is required, as most people consume more than enough fat and don't require additional fat in the form of milk, nor do adult men need to eat more beef, as this is likely to be turned into fat as well.

The other problem with milk is that like eggs and chicken it can be a source of *Salmonella* infection. In 1985, some 160,000 people became ill and several died in a massive outbreak of antimicrobial-resistant salmonellosis traced to pasteurized milk. This was in the USA (in Chicago), where if you did not get a bacterial infection you were liable to get a continuing low dose of antibiotics as a result of growth-promotion antibiotics given to cows. This might only be 50 micrograms a day, but over the milk-drinking life of a person, this can add up to quite a large amount.

Despite our ancestry as hunter–gatherers, we no longer need to eat large quantities of meat. (This in fact probably rarely happened, as it was more commonly gatherer–hunters, with more of the food coming from what could be gathered, with only the occasional successful hunt.) Animal protein is more likely to produce coronary artery thrombosis and heart attacks than fish and vegetable protein. Some evidence for why this might be was a finding that intestinal microbes metabolize L-carnitine, a nutrient found in red meat that promotes the development of atherosclerosis.

Fish Oil

During the war years of 1940–1945, shortages led to the government imposing food rationing, and giving supplements to children to ensure that they had an adequate diet. This in fact was a remarkable achievement, as not only did these prevent children from becoming malnourished but produced one of the best fed (in terms of health) generations of children ever. One of the supplements was cod liver oil, hated by children but spooned down us never the less. The purpose for this was that it was a high energy source food, full of fat-soluble vitamins, and one thing that could be done in a food-short Britain was to continue to catch fish.

While most of this was white fish (cod in particular), the liver of white fish contains omega-3 fatty acids, which have subsequently been found to have a protective effect on a number of medical conditions. An easier source of omega-3 is from the oily fishes – tuna, mackerel, herrings, trout and salmon, which contain the oil within their tissues and belly cavity.

Omega-3 has been found to reduce the risk of myocardial infarction by preventing cardiac arrhythmias, as well as being converted into resolvins, which reduce inflammation, a beneficial effect both on the cardiovascular system and in the prevention of arthritis. Several studies have also shown that the consumption of oily fish reduced the incidence of dementia. The recommendation is that 200–400 grams of oily fish are eaten twice a week.

Antioxidants

Another valuable protective component of food, along with dietary fibre, is found in the antioxidant properties of fruit and vegetables. Antioxidants protect cells against free radical damage produced by the production of oxygen during photosynthesis. Free radicals cause oxidation, so any antioxidants that are present are oxidized instead of cellular damage occurring. This both protects the cell and allows cellular damage to be repaired. The highest antioxidant levels are found in prunes, raisins, blueberries and blackberries. Although vegetables such as Brussels sprouts and broccoli contain lesser amounts, you eat more of them, so the same protective effects are achieved. Several vitamins are important antioxidants as well, but excess use, such as by vitamin supplementation, can cause adverse effects.

We are fortunate that the very first plants had to deal with the problem of photo-oxidation of chlorophyll when photosynthesis was developed, so they invented antioxidant systems that included compounds such as carotenoids. These were to protect the plant from the damage that excess oxygen would produce, so by selectively consuming these plant derivatives, we can similarly protect ourselves from the oxidation of our cells.

Carotenoids, as their name suggests, are found in carrots, but they are also contained in coloured fruits such as tomatoes, mangoes and pawpaws, as are other coloured antioxidants, such as anthocyanins. When these fruits are ripe they change colour from green to orange or red, or other colours, so attracting birds and animals to eat them and transfer the seeds in their droppings. It is likely then that the high levels of carotenes and other antioxidants found in the fruits of various plants have a dual role – as cell protectant antioxidants in the growing fruit, and as an attractant to animal dispersers of the fruit.

Mediterranean Diet

People living in the Mediterranean part of Europe, especially in Greece and Italy, have been found to live a long and healthy life, attributed to the food they eat. This is particularly high in fruit, vegetables and nuts, with fish rather than meat as the main protein constituent of the diet. Vegetable oil, particularly olive oil, is used rather than animal fat. This supports the earlier work done by Trowell and others, and the eating of a Mediterranean type diet is now often used as an expression of the ideal. Many people seeking a healthier lifestyle now make this diet their norm. A recent study of a sample of 4676 mid-to-older aged nurses taking part in the US Nurses' Health Study, which started in 1976, found that those living on a Mediterranean type diet had longer and healthier telomeres. Telomeres are the caps that protect the ends of chromosomes and prevent the loss of genetic information during cell division. This meant that there was less scrambling of the DNA with age, thus reducing the ageing process. As the authors, Crous-Bou *et al.*, concluded in a study reported in 2014: 'Greater adherence to the Mediterranean diet was significantly associated with longer leucocyte telomere length, a marker of biological aging'.

We need 20 essential amino acids to construct all the proteins in our bodies, but we can only manufacture 12 of them; the rest we must get from our food. Similarly, 13 vitamins are essential for all our life processes to be carried out, but we can only make two of them, vitamins D and B_7 (biotin). These need to be part of our diets although we might get help from one of our commonest gut bacteria, *Escherichia coli*, which can manufacture all of them with ease.

Preparing your own food not only allows you to include preferable constituents but to balance these to your individual needs, however many people take the easy way out. The fast-food industry at first provided a convenient source of food for the temporary visitor or for those in a hurry, but has grown into the regular food source of the mid and younger generations. This has now been joined by the pre-cooked ready meal, which just needs reheating. Unfortunately, these foods take no account of the individual's requirement in terms of protein, fat, carbohydrate and sugar, and are generally excessive in both sugar and salt. Sadly, fast foods in the form of burgers and chips have been exported to the rest of the world, so that the resultant obesity from their consumption has now become an international problem.

Obesity Promotion

What seems a complete irony is that while obesity, especially child-hood obesity, is now recognized as one of the most serious threats to human health, there is a proliferation of television programmes on food and cooking. Celebrity cooks vie with each other to produce the tastier meal, using excess salt, fat and sugar, at the same time often pro-pounding the health benefits of reducing these constituents. Even from a hygiene point of view these programmes set a bad example, for the cooks use bare hands and taste food from spoons, in complete contrast to the rest of the food industry, which requires protective clothing and gloves during food production. What they should be promoting is not only good food hygiene but also how to make meals more balanced, if perhaps less tasty.

In much of the developing world, especially Africa, the average meal is virtually the same, day in day out, yet in times when there is no food shortage, people develop healthy, strong bodies without becoming obese. In Africa, maize meal or cassava are the staple foods in much of the con-tinent, with a sauce to add some variety. There is no effort to make the food tastier and, as a result, obesity is not a problem.

If the present rate of obesity continues to increase, it is anticipated that there will be a decline in the expectation of life, as well as an increased burden on the health services. It seems that we don't need microbes or parasites to produce disease, we are doing this ourselves. We are selecting against ourselves rather than disease doing this for us.

Food Poisoning

The food we eat is also a ready source of nourishment for disease-producing organisms, and food poisoning is a common problem. Major outbreaks are notified, but many minor ones do not get reported to the authorities and those in the home might pass as a minor disruption of family life. The onset is sudden with fever and vomiting, with or without diarrhoea, in a group of persons that have shared the same meal. Sometimes there is a subnormal temperature and a fall in blood pressure, with the person collapsing or feeling faint. The incubation period is short and sufficiently precise that the type of organism can often be determined – if it is under 6 hours then it is likely to be a *Staphylococcus*, while if it is over 6 hours it is more likely to be a *Salmonella*.

Staphylococcal food poisoning results from toxin produced by the bacteria, so the food may be adequately cooked but was infected during preparation or through poor storage. This is normally by a food handler with an infected lesion on the fingers, or unhygienic practices such as transferring bacteria from the nose.

Salmonella food poisoning results from infection of the animal in the living state, such as occurs in chickens and their eggs, and also from contaminating processes in the slaughter of animals, particularly cattle and pigs. There has been considerable improvement since the 1990s, when large numbers of chickens were found to be infected. However in some parts of the world, such as Adelaide, Australia, 38.8% of chicken samples tested were found to be positive for *Salmonella* in 2008 (BioPortfolio.com, 21 December 2014). In the UK, the Food Standards Agency reported 1562 food and environmental contaminant incidents in 2013, 30% of which were due to *Salmonella*. The main organisms were *S. enteritidis* and *S. typhimurium*. It is, therefore, imperative that any poultry or fresh meat is properly cooked, with particular care taken when cooking whole chickens, as sometimes the inside is not adequately cooked when the outside is quite brown. It is often preferable to divide the carcase into smaller sections and cook these separately.

There are other forms of food poisoning such as that from *Vibrio parahaemolyticus*, which is more commonly associated with seafood or food that has been washed with contaminated seawater, or the more serious *Clostridium botulinum*, which can occur from improperly prepared home-preserves. Such is the potency of the toxin from *C. botulinum* that it has been considered for use as a method of germ warfare.

In 401 BC, the Greek commander Xenephon noticed that his soldiers had become violently ill from consuming what was called 'mad honey'. This is made by bees collecting the nectar of rhododendrons, which contains a toxin that blocks nerve impulses. When the Greeks were invaded by the Romans, they placed pots of this honey in tempting places, making the attacking soldiers ill and easy prey for the defending Greeks.

There are specific forms of fish poisoning caused by toxins, which are either present in fish or shellfish when they partially decompose or can result if the gut contents are not removed immediately. Buying whole fish that have been kept on ice can often produce diarrhoea, as the gut of the fish is left intact and some decomposition may have taken place, so that even when the gut is removed it has already leaked into the rest of the fish.

Campylobacter

Another infection associated with the consumption of food is that produced by *Campylobacter*, which is increasing for similar reasons to infection by *Salmonella* (discussed below). Infection by *Campylobacter* presents more as a self-limiting attack of diarrhoea within 4–7 days, but more serious infections with blood in the stool can occur, with a similar presentation to bacillary dysentery. Domestic animals, including poultry, pigs, sheep, cats and dogs, are reservoirs of the organism, and consumption of or close association with these animals is responsible for much of the transmission. Faecal contamination of unpasteurized milk and untreated water also leads to infection, with children more often the victims than adults. In December 2014, the Food Standards Agency raised concern about *Campylobacter*, finding 70% of chickens taken from supermarkets shelves positive for the bacterium and 18% above the highest contamination levels.

Salmonella and food contamination

Salmonella infection has now become the most important cause of food-borne disease in the world, mainly due to globalization and the search for profit by the food industry, at the expense of the health of the general public. Surprisingly, low-dose antibiotics have been found to improve meat production, so they have been used extensively by the agricultural industry, resulting in the development of drug-resistant *Salmonella*. An example is *S. typhimurium* phage type DT104, which is now a globally multi-drug-resistant organism. The European Union banned the practice of feeding low-dose antibiotics in 1999, but it still continues in the USA and in other parts of the world from which we obtain meat.

While antibiotic enhancement of meat production is no longer practised in the home industry, the globalization of food supply makes control almost impossible, with instances of the failure of national mechanisms to check quality and safety. Such is the lure of profits that food producers will take short cuts and risk the health and often the lives of consumers, especially those of the young and the elderly. Buying locally – if the product genuinely is produced locally, as some local producers just unpack produce from a central distributor – is a precaution that can be taken, as is avoiding altogether such foods as meat, which is the main culprit. There are many advantages of a vegetarian diet and this is certainly one of them.

If it is not the food item that is doing the travelling then it is the widespread movement of people through tourism, immigration or the deployment of workforces that has exposed people to unfamiliar foods and those whose safety is in doubt. Ensuring that items are freshly cooked is the best precaution and often the smaller restaurant, where this can be seen to be done, is safer than the large hotel that needs to present an extensive menu, meaning that unused food may be stored and put out on more than one occasion.

It is surprising that people should consider taking short cuts or adulterating foods in the search for profits, knowing that they may be endangering the lives of others and when they also need to eat, but sadly such is the ever-present reality. With food, not only do we have to contend with disease organisms that compromise our health but unscrupulous humans as well.

Cancer

The daughter of one of the five illegitimate children of Juan Duarte and Juana Ibarguren fortunately had sufficient charisma and good looks to become an actress. As well as being on the stage, she was a well-known voice on the radio, abilities that brought her to the attention of Colonel Juan Perón in 1944, to become his second wife in the following year. Juan Perón became the president of Argentina in 1946, but Eva, or Evita, as she was more popularly known, never forgot her humble roots. In 1948, she formed the Eva Perón foundation, with which she built hospitals, schools, orphanages and homes for the aged, endearing herself to the masses, who she called 'los descamisados' (the shirtless ones). She was also a prominent feminist, largely responsible for getting the women's suffrage law passed, but at the height of her popularity and only 33 years of age, she died from breast cancer.

Even after death she remained a symbol of the working classes, and when Perón was deposed in 1955 her body was taken to Italy, where it remained for 16 years. When Perón died in 1974 it was brought back to be placed in a crypt next to him, but 2 years later the military junta, keen to try to extinguish all traces of Peronism, removed the bodies. After further years of wandering, the much travelled remains of Evita were eventually laid to rest in the Duarte family crypt in Rocoleta cemetery in Buenos Aires.

Cancer Incidence

Breast cancer is the commonest cause of cancer in women and the commonest cancer in both sexes in Europe. Only lung cancer kills more people from neoplastic disease in the world. Compared with several of the other cancers, breast cancer remains an enigma, for despite all the research done no strong association with any causal factor has been found, except for a genetic predisposition in a small group of unfortunate women who have either the *BRCA1* or *BRCA2* genes, or two variants of the *KLF4* gene. Breastfeeding for a substantial period has a protective effect, but despite this being universally practised in developing countries, breast cancer remains an important cause of mortality in Africa and Asia, as well as in the more developed sector of the world.

The country with the highest death rate from breast cancer is, surprisingly, Saint Kitts and Nevis, at 36.1 cases per 100,000; the second highest is in another Caribbean group of islands, Antigua and Barbuda at 29.8. At the other extreme is also an island nation, Samoa, with a rate of only 1.5 cases per 100,000, with Mongolia second lowest at 3.8. In Europe, Bosnia/Herzegovina has the lowest rate of 13.3 deaths per 100,000, with Finland next at 16.3. Even in two countries that share similar racial and geographical characteristics, Australia and New Zealand, the rate in Australia is 18.2 and that in New Zealand 21.5. There are no features that indicate why these rates should be so different in such disparate parts of the world, and the enigma of breast cancer causation continues.

There is a very remote indication that breast cancer had its origins with the very first mammals, the multituberculates, monotreme-like rodents that originated before the dinosaurs some 250 million years ago, but then went extinct some 30 million years BP. They were the first to develop mammary tissues and in so doing attracted a virus infection that is revealed today in the mouse mammary tumour virus. This has served as an experimental model for human breast cancer, but so far has not been found to be causal of the human disease.

A similar situation is found in males with prostate cancer, which was the fourth most common cancer in the world in 2012 according to Cancer Research UK estimates. This disease, however, is age related, and when post-mortems are done on elderly males, most of them are found to have some degree of prostate cancer. Intriguingly, dogs have been found to be very good at sniffing out prostate cancer sufferers, but due to the inevitability of this age-related condition, the use of this method needs to be carefully evaluated. Recent research has shown that vitamin D inhibits growth of cancer cells in the prostate and the next most common cancer, bowel cancer, so might have value in preventing these conditions.

Bowel cancer is the third most common cancer in the world and has been on the increase, as a study by Parkin *et al.*, reported in 1984 but based on data collected in 1975, estimated it to be the fourth most common cancer at that time. Parkin's study also found that stomach cancer was the leading cancer; this is still a common problem in Asia, but now has become fifth in rank, largely due to the increase in lung, breast and bowel cancers.

Cancer is a different disease process from that produced by parasites, in that it is caused by cells in the body that continue to proliferate and spread throughout the body; in effect, the body attacks itself. Normal cells are programmed to kill themselves when they have outlived their usefulness, and it is this process that goes wrong, leading to the cells continuing to divide and reproduce. There is generally not one factor that leads to this happening, except in a few now fortunately rare occupational cancers, such as the scrotal cancer of chimney sweeps and those cancers suffered by the early workers with X-rays or asbestos.

Most cancers are age related, so that in Western countries there is a 1:4 chance of dying from cancer in old age. Other cancers have strong causal factors, such as cigarette smoking and lung cancer, but many seem to have a range of causes and it is only after a tipping point has been reached that the cancerous growth proliferates in its unstoppable manner.

Cancer Prevention

Fortunately there are some preventive actions that can be taken, such as not smoking or not drinking excessive amounts of alcohol, but perhaps the one that is of benefit in preventing most cancers is dietary modification. Bowel cancer is potentiated by irritant substances remaining in the intestines, so a rapid transit time, as is produced by a high fibre content of the diet, prevents this from happening. Fruit and vegetables not only have a fibre content but also contain antioxidants, which facilitate programmed cell death, so have a preventive effect on cancer cells of many different kinds.

Although we have a full complement of genes, many have several different actions while not all are turned on. This is particularly affected by nutritional factors, especially certain vitamins. The mechanism by which genes are turned on or off is called methylation, with some genes turned on by methylation and some turned off. This offers particular hope in the prevention of cancer with, for example, the connection between the gene *PITX2* and breast cancer. In a study in Germany, 90% of women with low methylation of the gene were found to be safe from contracting breast cancer, while those with high methylation carried a greater risk. There were several factors that produced this methylation, with some of them specific to the individual, so it might well be that customized cancer prevention and treatment will be the way forward.

Smoking is such a powerful gene methylater in many different conditions that it produces hypermethylation. In contrast, drinking green tea inhibits methylation of the genes that protect against colon, prostate and oesophageal cancers.

Viruses have been found to be the cause, or an associated cause, of several cancers, one of the most common being primary liver cancer. This is the main cause of cancer in Africa and the sixth most common in the world. There is, however, a strong association with hepatitis B infection, so now that there is an effective vaccine, which is being given routinely to children in many countries, we can hope to see a considerable decrease in this unpleasant disease.

There is similar hope for cervical cancer, which is the seventh most common cancer in the world, mainly because of its preponderance in developing countries. In Africa it kills more women than breast cancer. The main cause is the human papilloma virus, for which there is a vaccine. By vaccinating girls before they become sexually active, it is hoped to considerably reduce the burden of this distressing form of cancer.

Viruses probably are associated with, although not the main cause of, several other cancers. A virus was discovered jointly by Drs Epstein and Barr, and for a long time it was a virus looking for a disease, until it was found to be the cause of infectious mononucleosis. It now seems that the Epstein–Barr virus (EBV) might also be a causal factor in non-Hodgkin's lymphoma and nasopharyngeal cancer, as well as in the complex aetiology of Burkitt's lymphoma.

Denis Burkitt (1911–1993) was part of the brilliant group of doctors at Makerere University in Uganda that made such a contribution to health and health services in the 1960s. Hugh Trowell has already been mentioned in Chapter 15, but in addition there was Maurice King, who developed the Primary Health Care System, David Morley, who promoted Maternal and Child Health Care, and David Bradley, who did pioneer research into schistosomiasis and leishmaniasis. Denis Burkitt was a surgeon but he did one of the most original of epidemiological studies.

Noticing that a childhood tumour affecting the jaw and face seemed to be more common than at first realized, he set out to collect every case that had been identified. At first, it was thought that all the cases were restricted to sub-Saharan Africa, but later cases were also found in Papua New Guinea. Putting these all on a map, there appeared to be a close association with the distribution of malaria. EBV was later identified, and it was thought that chronic malaria reduced the body's defences, so allowing the lymphoma to take hold. Hopefully, with the control of malaria, there will be a decrease in this distressing tumour.

Some larger parasites, mainly by their presence as constant irritants, increase the likelihood of developing cancer. The trematode worm *Schistosoma haematobium* causes a common disease in Africa and Arabia, and will often cause cancer of the bladder, while another flatworm, *Clonorchis sinensis*, which lives in the gall bladder, is responsible for many cases of cholangiocarcinoma, particularly in China and South-east Asia, where it is mainly found.

There is, therefore, hope of reducing several cancers by treating these diseases or by vaccination where there is a viral cause. Sadly, the common afflictions of breast and prostate cancer have only yielded a few clues as to how they may be reduced.

As the majority of cancers occur after the reproductive age, natural selection will have no effect on their prevalence, while disease selection will do likewise, except in individual cases, like that of Evita, to whom it gave something like martyr status.

Climate Change and Population Movements

17

We live in a changing world, and the dual processes of climate change and urbanization will bring us into greater conflict with disease. The change in climate due to global warming will be from an increase in temperature and from changes in weather patterns, with more storms and flooding.

One of the largest weather systems is the El Niño southern oscillation, which can reverse or become severely disrupted, bringing heavy rain and flooding when no rain is normally expected and drought conditions during the rainy season. Countries in South America, South-east Asia and Oceania are mostly affected, but some disruption is felt all over the world. In the northern hemisphere, the occurrence of revolving tropical storms – cyclones, typhoons or hurricanes, depending on where in the world they occur – appear to be increasing in frequency and ferocity, bringing disruption and damage, leading to an increase in diseases that flourish in such conditions, such as diarrhoeal infections.

Effects on Diseases

Outbreaks of plague in Ecuador appear to have an association with El Niño (the boy child) – referring to the Christ child, as it normally occurs around Christmas time – while its converse, La Niña (the girl child) has had an association with the last four pandemics of influenza. This is considered to be due to a cooling of ocean surface temperatures that takes place before La Niña, altering the migration of birds, so bringing them into unexpected contact with domestic poultry and animals.

Increase in temperature has the potential to expand the range of infections that are normally constrained by temperature, such as malaria. This has led to speculation that malaria could once again become established in Europe and North America, where it occurred in former times (see Chapter 18), but this is unlikely to happen. A good example is Australia, where much of the country lies within the tropical region and the main malaria vector *Anopheles farauti* – the same as in New Guinea and Solomon Islands – is present, yet control methods have eradicated the parasite and continued surveillance has prevented its reintroduction.

A more serious problem is in areas of highlands within tropical countries, such as found in East Africa and South America, where the temperature at higher altitudes limits the height at which malaria is found. Studies conducted in Ethiopia and Kenya have discovered that malaria has progressively occurred at higher altitudes and that there is a wider fluctuation of temperature, thus increasing the likelihood of epidemic malaria breaking out in people that have no immunity. Other diseases transmitted by mosquitoes, such as Japanese encephalitis and Rift Valley fever, are also likely to increase.

While global warming will favour the mosquito, it has been shown that increased water temperature will have an adverse effect on the snail, in which the intermediate stages of *Schistosoma mansoni* develop. As the water becomes warmer, the number of suitable habitats will decrease, reducing the chance of people coming into contact with this infection.

Leishmaniasis is an established disease in southern Europe, producing indolent skin ulcers that can persist for many years if not treated. Favourable conditions could extend the range of the vector sandfly (*Phlebotomus*) further north; however, the *Phlebotomus* species concerned already has a range greater than the pathogen and the main reservoir of infection is in dogs, which are widely distributed, so there is no reason to expect this disease to increase its extent in Europe. In contrast, *Ixodes ricinus*, the main vector of Lyme disease and tick-borne encephalitis (TBE) in Europe, has already extended its range into more northerly latitudes of Scandinavia and higher altitudes of the Czech Republic, so there is likely to be an increase in these diseases. Also, the prolonged season could intensify transmission in areas where infection is already a problem.

While much of the concern for an increase in disease due to global warming has been expressed in Western countries, it is more likely that most of the effect will be concentrated in the poorer regions of the world, with an increase in vector-borne and diarrhoeal diseases, malnutrition and the health problems that follow natural disasters.

Urbanization

During the last century, the majority of the world population lived in rural areas, but with the steady movement of people to cities, more people now live in urban areas. This has brought with it the problems of slum conditions and resultant ill health, mainly from the diseases of poor hygiene. Conversely, the population is more concentrated, making it easier for health services to be provided for a greater number of people but, unfortunately, resource limitations prevent many countries from doing this. An unexpected consequence of urbanization is linked to the problem of global warming and the rise in sea level that will take place. Thirteen of the 20 major conurbations are at sea level, with Bangladesh, China, India and Egypt the countries most affected. Some 550 million urban Asians were at risk of flooding in 2010, but this is expected to rise to 760 million by 2025. A further danger is that from earthquakes and tsunamis, meaning that there is now the potential for loss of life on a scale never seen before.

Another feature of urbanization is the increase in convenience stores and fast-food outlets, which takes place at a greater rate with collections of people. The problem of obesity has already been mentioned, so it is likely that increasing urbanization will go hand in hand with increasing obesity and all the health problems associated with this.

Population Movements

Population movements of a different kind have resulted in refugees who, due to disruption of their normal way of life, loss of important family members and poverty from the loss of possessions, as well as the psychological damage that occurs, have become more susceptible to disease. Some are even resettled into areas that bring them into closer contact with infectious diseases, as illustrated by the example of sleeping sickness in the Mishamo refugee settlement in Tanzania mentioned in Chapter 4. Sometimes misguided help makes the situation worse, such as happened when water storage jars were given to refugees settled along the Thai border during the Cambodian crisis. These proved to be ideal breeding places for *Aedes* mosquitoes so that, together with the concentrations of people, there were large outbreaks of dengue.

Local migrations from one country to a neighbouring country for trade or to visit relatives can risk the health of individuals or families. In much of South-east Asia borders generally follow ridges of high ground which, by their nature, are inaccessible and generally contain remnants of forest. Mosquitoes inhabit these forests and, as a result, malaria is more intense along these borders, making it six times as likely for people to catch malaria than if they had not travelled. This is a complex process (called forest border malaria), with the added complication of illegal cutting of timber, trade in narcotics and, sometimes, insurgents, all increasing the malaria problem and the difficulties of trying to do something about it. People often sleep in the temporary logging camps, and encouraging them to take insecticide-treated mosquito nets (ITNs) with them is one thing that can be done.

Travel, though, is essential and if our ancestors had not travelled in the first place, the human species would probably not have become what it is. This was a very dangerous passage, as can be seen from the limited amount of genetic variation that resulted. One can be certain that the journey was hampered by diseases similar to the examples above. There would have been direct competition between disease selection and natural selection but, fortunately for our species, natural selection won.

Disappeared and Emergent Diseases

18

European Malaria

Malaria got its name from the Italian for bad air ('mala aria') as this was thought to be how it was transmitted. It was a particular problem in the Pontine Marshes (a reclaimed area of marshland in central Italy) up to the middle part of the last century when concerted efforts were made to eradicate the disease. Corsica was one of the last parts of Europe to be cleared of malaria and became a trial ground for using insecticides on a large scale, leading to the global malaria eradication programme.

In Shakespeare's time malaria was endemic in England, where it was called the ague. It was caused by the less serious form *Plasmodium vivax*, which can persist in the liver, thus allowing it to be present in the blood during the next summer, when a fresh batch of *Anopheles* mosquitoes would have hatched. Shakespeare had looked forward to his new sovereign, James I, coming to the throne and, ironically, it was malaria that was to cause James's demise. The King lived until he was 59, but in the last years of his reign the Duke of Buckingham, in league with the then Prince Charles, took over most of the powers of the kingdom.

When Prince Charles became King, it was to lead to the civil war that was to devastate the nation. Charles died from the executioner's axe, while his adversary, Oliver Cromwell, succumbed to malaria. It was while Cromwell was campaigning in Ireland that his illness started, and he died in London a month later. Even in death though, his body was not allowed to lie in peace, as the vengeful Charles II had it exhumed and hung from the gallows at Tyburn. After it had been there for some time the head was removed and stuck on a pole on the top of Westminster Hall, to remain there until the end of Charles's reign.

Although we are now free of malaria, the *Anopheles* mosquitoes are still with us. The main culprit, *A. maculipennis*, has now been found to be a complex of at least seven species, marked by many different biological traits, although their outward appearances are identical. As mentioned in

Chapter 17, there is the potential for malaria to take hold again in Britain, but this is unlikely even if global warming should produce a marked increase in temperature. Also, some of the members of the *A. maculipennis* complex have changed their feeding habits, preferring cows to humans, so you are more likely to find the mosquito in cattle sheds than in the home.

Malaria was also a problem in Holland but died out due to the demise of the *Anopheles* mosquito vector, which particularly bred along the course of the River Rhine. Many years ago, I met an entomologist who for his PhD tried to find out the reason why the mosquito had died out – because if it were to return, it could be a vector of malaria again. He spent a long time looking for the reason, with many suggestions that he worked through one by one, until finally he came to the conclusion that the mosquito could no longer breed in the Rhine because it had become too polluted!

The English Sweat

When Henry VII landed from France on 7 August 1485 before the Battle of Bosworth, one of his mercenary soldiers had an illness that later became called the English Sweat. It was mentioned before the battle, but when Henry reached London on 28 August, an epidemic broke out that caused high mortality. The disease was quite distinct from the plague as there was no bubo or rash, and produced a high sweating fever that was rapidly fatal.

A second epidemic occurred in 1507, but with fewer fatalities, and then there was a third epidemic in 1517, which was particularly severe in Oxford and Cambridge, where half the population are said to have died.

The fourth epidemic in 1528 was devastating. It started in London and spread throughout the whole country, but spared Scotland, then crossed to the continent, ravaging north and eastern Europe where there was a high mortality. It then disappeared completely from continental Europe but returned again to England in 1551, when a good account of the disease was given by the physician John Kaye (but not using his old English):

> There was a sudden onset with severe apprehension, followed by cold shivers, giddiness, headache and severe pain in the back of the neck, shoulders and limbs. After this initial cold stage there was the hot stage of sweating, delirium, palpitations and pain in the chest, but never any rash. It could be fatal in as short as 2–3 hours after the first symptoms, but normally this happened between 12–24 hours. Those that survived for 24 hours normally recovered completely. Surprisingly it affected the richer classes, the poor hardly at all and children and infants never. It then disappeared completely and has never returned.

There has been much speculation as to what the 'English Sweat' was, but there are no symptom complexes that match this description. The very short illness and high fatality are unique, and why it completely disappeared, or where it came from in the first place remain a mystery.

Between 1718 and 1861 there was a similar but less fatal disease in France called the Picardy sweat. There have also been mentions of other diseases, such as the 'New Disease', of Elizabethan England that do not seem to fit any that we are familiar with, so new infections do appear out of the blue from time to time.

Eradication Programmes

The last case of smallpox was in October 1977 and the World Health Organization (WHO) certified the eradication of smallpox on 9 December 1979. This had been a triumph of medical prevention using a highly effective vaccine and dedicated teams, working even in wartime situations. Controversially, live cultures of smallpox still remain in secure laboratories in the USA and Russia but, providing these are never allowed to escape, smallpox as a disease will never be seen again.

There are other pox diseases, the most important of which is monkeypox (see Chapter 5), and for a time after smallpox had been eradicated there was concern that this could take its place. It is, however, a rare disease, localized to the tropical rainforest areas of West and Central Africa, with occasional human cases, but the secondary attack rate is much lower than that of smallpox so is unlikely to increase to epidemic levels.

Although not a human disease, rinderpest was declared eradicated on 14 October 2010 after no cases had appeared for 9 years. Its importance has been mentioned earlier (Chapter 12) in terms of human suffering due to the devastation of cattle on which many tribes were dependent.

The similarity between the measles virus and the rinderpest virus means that measles could be eliminated, and efforts have been made, particularly in the Americas, to do this, with the gratifying result that on 29 April 2015, the Americas became the first WHO region to eradicate the disease. Unfortunately, little progress has been made in the rest of the world.

The WHO set out to eliminate poliomyelitis by the turn of the century, but this target has had to be continually revised, although good progress is being made, with many parts of the world completely free of the disease. In 2012, there were only 223 cases of wild polio, 122 in Nigeria, 58 in Pakistan, 37 in Afghanistan, five in Chad and one in Niger, but by 2013, the total number had risen to 385. Several of the affected areas are conflict zones and religious intolerance has led to setbacks.

Guinea worm, which causes dracunculiasis, is the longest subcutaneous parasitic worm ever known and is transmitted by the accidental consumption of copepods (*Cyclops* and others) in infected well water.

An extensive programme of protecting wells from water washing back into them has been hugely successful in almost eradicating this horrific parasite. In 2013, only 148 cases were found, 76% of them in South Sudan.

Yaws (see Chapter 13), a disfiguring infection of skin and bone, has been eradicated from most of the world using programmes of long-acting penicillin injections, but cases still persist in remote areas of Côte d'Ivoire, Ghana, Togo, Cameroon, Central African Republic, Democratic Republic of the Congo, Indonesia, Timor-Leste, Papua New Guinea, Solomon Islands and Vanuatu. It is mainly a case of finding these often hidden cases that is preventing the complete elimination of this disease.

A programme to eliminate lymphatic filariasis is in operation in the tropical regions of the world using mass drug administration and insecticide-treated mosquito nets, but it will be a lengthy process to reduce the disease as the adult worm has a long life history. However, some 6.6 million new cases had been prevented by October 2008.

Leprosy, the disease of antiquity, is declining worldwide due to careful search-and-find teams and follow-up treatment programmes. It will be many years before the scars of this awful condition are removed from the world, but its decline in all countries of the world except for central and southern Africa, Madagascar and the Indian subcontinent makes this now a disappearing disease.

New Diseases

In contrast to this picture of hope and freedom from disease is another of new diseases that appear quite unexpectedly. Many of these are viral diseases and those transmitted by mosquitoes make up a considerable number. There have been at least 118 of these diseases, some affecting very limited areas, such as Ross River fever in Australia and New Zealand or St Louis encephalitis in the USA, while others have become more widespread, such as West Nile fever, which expanded out of its usual area of prevalence to produce epidemics in the USA and Canada.

Then there was the 2001–2008 epidemic of Chicungunya, normally a disease of East Africa, but in January 2001 cases were discovered in Indonesia, thousands of miles away from its usual focus. The epidemic really took off in 2006, with cases in Malaysia, Comoro Islands, Seychelles, Mauritius and a particularly severe epidemic in the island of Réunion, which with its dengue-like symptoms of fever and arthritis almost brought the island to a standstill. From here, cases were carried back to Europe and in August 2007 local transmission took place in the Emilia Romagna region of north-east Italy, from a person who had been infected in India. This was due to the presence of *Aedes albopictus*, now widespread in many parts of the world, making the spread of other, and perhaps more serious, arboviral infections a considerable matter of concern.

In 2012 a new disease appeared in Saudi Arabia caused by a corona virus and since called Middle East respiratory syndrome (MERS). The first cases were contracted from close contact with camels but it appears to have been a disease of bats which was transmitted to camels in the distant past. The symptoms are fever, cough and shortness of breath and, in the severe case, the development of pneumonia, with a 36% mortality rate. Over 1000 cases have so far been reported from 26 countries. Transmission is now mainly due to close personal contact, with health staff and those looking after sick relatives at particular risk. Infection can still, however, be contracted from camels, so the handling of camels or visiting camel markets are risk factors as well as eating improperly cooked camel meat or drinking camel milk.

As well as the rodent-associated diseases previously mentioned, one emerging disease is that produced by the hantavirus. This causes two differing clinical syndromes, haemorrhagic fever with renal syndrome found in the Balkans, eastern Russia, China and Korea, and hantavirus pulmonary syndrome in North and South America. Transmission is thought to be respiratory, from an aerosol of rodent excreta, so precautions need to be taken in areas where rats and field rodents are commonly found. Fortunately, human-to-human infection does not occur.

The importance of close association with animals, and infection jumping from one species to another, has been extensively covered in Chapter 12, but it will always remain a potential threat. While contact with animals is the main method of transmission, their consumption is another possibility, and the fascination by tourists in sampling exotic animals for the table might have consequences that they did not anticipate.

It is a mistake to think that the communicable diseases have been beaten, as there is good evidence that old diseases are expanding into areas where they were not normally found and new diseases are appearing. This happened in antiquity and will happen again in the future. Infecting organisms are evolving and finding different methods to express themselves in a range of new diseases that will be our future lot.

The Future

19

Obesity

When I first started working in developing countries, the main problem was not so much how to control disease but how to overcome the poverty and poor nutrition that made people, especially children, more susceptible to communicable diseases. Poverty, lack of education, ignorance and resentment at applying simple preventive strategies were our main problems. Finding enough food was the continual struggle that families went through, and in countries in which the weather followed a seasonal pattern, drought and starvation were an ever-present threat. It seems almost inconceivable that one of the major problems of the world now is obesity, in particular child obesity, and it is not just in the more developed world but in the developing world as well.

There is still the big divide, with a large segment of the population in poverty and generally underweight. Sadly, those that have managed to lift themselves out of poverty have adopted the poor nutritional diet of Western nations, so obesity has become common among them.

The World Health Organization (WHO) reports that worldwide obesity has doubled since 1980, with 60% of the world's population living in countries where overweight and obesity kill more people than underweight. Some 35% of adults aged 20 years and over were overweight in 2008, totalling more than 1.4 billion, with more overweight women than men. If these figures are not startling enough, more than 40 million children under the age of 5 years were overweight or obese in 2012, indicating the rapidly increasing problem in the future.

Obesity leads to an increase in heart disease, type 2 diabetes, cancer and osteoarthritis, and the US government reckons the excess cost of obesity to the health services was US$1429 per obese person or US$147 billion in total in 2008. More than one third (35%) or 78.6 million US adults are obese.

Susceptibility to heart disease has a genetic component, which is influenced by a geographical trend. People in northern Europe are more likely to get heart attacks than those in southern Europe, while Asians are less likely than Europeans. Africans, Polynesians and Melanesians also have this susceptibility, but on their traditional diet this is not revealed. However, once they change to a Western style diet of hamburgers and chips their risk of developing early heart attacks increases rapidly. One can, therefore, postulate that there will be a considerable increase in heart disease in some developing countries, especially in urban areas where fast-food outlets proliferate.

The enormity of the problem is only superseded by the speed at which obesity is increasing, meaning that it will be the major cause of ill health in the future. What is so tragic is that it is all totally preventable with a reduction in fats and refined sugars in the diet, an increase in the fruit and vegetable component and an increase in exercise. Even small changes can be beneficial, walking for half an hour each day and limiting the amount we eat will gradually reduce weight and lead to a healthier lifestyle.

Influenza

Between 2009 and 2011 there was the pandemic of influenza called swine flu because of its origin in pigs in Mexico. At first it was thought this might be the massive pandemic that experts in the field were anticipating, but it turned out that the strain concerned, A/H1N1, was an original strain of influenza. This was why it predominantly affected the younger age groups, as the older generation had met A/H1N1 before. Antigenic shift either of the H or N components has occurred at regular intervals, leading to the pandemics of the past, as mentioned in Chapter 10, so a new shift is overdue, and a resultant pandemic of global proportions likely. Influenza has been one of the greatest killers, with the mortality of the 1918 epidemic one of the largest in the history of humankind. We are prepared for such an epidemic as never before with vaccines and antiviral drugs, but it is still likely to produce a substantial mortality, especially in regions of the world where access is difficult.

Ebola

The epidemic of Ebola that has raged in West Africa demonstrates what can happen to a normally controllable disease that gets out of hand. Ebola has been known for some time, and cases, generally in expatriates unfortunate enough to become infected, were evacuated under strict barrier nursing conditions to high-security treatment facilities. This pattern of occurrence suggested that Ebola was endemic in the community and that only those without any previous experience of infection were susceptible.

An animal source was thought to be the reservoir, as in Lassa fever, with bats the most likely culprits.

The first epidemic occurred in a localized area and although most people died, the area was sufficiently isolated, with little movement to surrounding areas, so it was contained. What has been different this time has been the movement of people and the continued contact, so that the epidemic has increased exponentially. Close contact is difficult to avoid, especially in crowded market places, on buses and visiting neighbours, while even after the person has recovered the semen remains infective for some 10 weeks, so sexual transmission has also occurred. Hopefully people will be more aware in the future of what can happen and act more rapidly to seal off the area and treat the infected.

Antimicrobial Resistance

While epidemics will call for emergency action, a more intractable problem is that of antimicrobial resistance. The first antibiotic was the sulfonamide Prontosil in 1932, developed from a synthetic coal-tar dye. Its active ingredient was discovered to be sulfanilamide, and this led to the production of many different sulfa preparations that saved the lives of thousands of people, including Winston Churchill, in the pre-war and early years of World War II. When methods were finally developed for the mass production of penicillin, it largely superseded the sulfonamides, as it was more effective and did not have the side effects that were severe in patients with a sensitivity to the sulfonamides. Unfortunately, soon after its introduction in 1940 resistance appeared, with the result that new antibiotics, such as the tetracyclines, were produced. Some organisms then developed resistance to these broad-spectrum antibiotics, and it has been a continuous race to produce new ones ever since.

Fungi and algae have been protecting themselves from bacteria for millennia with the production of natural antibiotics, the same as we have synthesized for use in the treatment of human infections. However, bacteria developed resistance to these natural antibiotics, which they have since carried on their genes. When a team of scientists analysed bacteria from the permafrost of the Yukon in Canada that were at least 30,000 years old, they found that they were able to resist the naturally produced antibiotics from bread mould. While these ancient genes might have initiated the process, it has been the continuous drug pressure exerted by the medical and agricultural use of antibiotics that has accelerated the development of resistance.

A further problem has been the use of antibiotics in the food industry for the growth promotion of animals. While this is now less of a problem in Europe since the practice was banned in 1999, it still continues in the USA. Small amounts of these antibiotics are retained in meat, eggs and milk, so that over many years they can accumulate in the body, which is especially important in children. This not only helps to induce the development of resistance but can also damage the immune system, as mentioned in Chapter 14, and lead to obesity (Chapter 15).

Staphylococcus aureus has been problematic from the start, developing resistance to each of the penicillins (and other types of antibiotics) soon after they were developed, leading to methicillin-resistant *S. aureus*, commonly known as MRSA. This is now a serious hospital infection and although many people carry this organism as a commensal, often in the nose, it is in hospital that serious wound infections result.

Recently, a strain of MRSA identical to that in humans has been found in cattle, particularly in their dung, indicating that this might have been where the resistant strain originally came from or, if not, that it is now an additional source of that strain. This might have developed from the use of low-dose antibiotics to improve meat yield, as mentioned in Chapter 15.

Reliance on combating MRSA has depended on cleanliness and the use of antiseptics, especially by attendant staff and visitors, and is similar to the pre-antibiotic era methods developed by Semmelweis and Lister. These can be surprisingly effective if carried out diligently. A similar problem arose in the 1960s when the availability of new antibiotics had been exhausted. The brave decision was taken to halt the use of antibiotics – except under strict supervision to those with life-threatening conditions – and rely upon cleanliness and antisepsis. In time, the resistant strain of the organism was replaced by original strains that conferred other advantages once the blanket use of antibiotics had been removed. It may be necessary to use the same strategy again.

Antibiotics, especially those with a broad spectrum of action, kill off microbes that are not the cause of the target infection. When respiratory and other infections are treated with antibiotics, they also kill off the normal gut flora, making the person susceptible to intestinal infections, particularly from *Salmonella* and *Campylobacter*. Many of these are also antibiotic resistant, leading to a serious problem in how to treat the patient.

The excessive use of antibiotics in treating infection, or the more questionable practice of giving antibiotic cover where no infection has actually occurred, as is practised frequently after operations, has allowed organisms that are not normally pathogens to develop, such as *Clostridium difficile*. This produces a pseudomembranous colitis with prolonged diarrhoea and fulminating toxic megacolon. Patients in hospital with other conditions are particularly susceptible. Fortunately, a new experimental treatment that tries to replace the gut bacteria killed off by antibiotics, using the transplantation of faecal microbiota, is showing considerable promise. While this has so far only been tried for *C. difficile*, it has established the principle that replacing these bacteria from a healthy donor could be used to treat a range of bacterial and allergic conditions. This would seem to be the case for ulcerative colitis, as it is a bowel condition, but might also be effective for other allergies, as it is mainly the loss of useful gut bacteria that is the problem.

Other organisms that have developed antibiotic resistance are those that cause tuberculosis (TB), gonorrhoea, typhoid and cholera. The cause of TB, *Mycobacterium tuberculosis*, has in some places become completely resistant to treatment – especially in parts of Russia – so that there are now no alternative medicaments. Such cases have to be kept in fully sterile conditions with barrier nursing to prevent them spreading further.

The treatment of cholera is by the replacement of fluid and electrolytes, as discussed in Chapter 9, and antibiotics are not required. So why has resistance developed? Antibiotics provide a limited prophylactic value, but simple precautions, as mentioned in Chapter 9, are perfectly adequate. However, such is the hysteria during a cholera epidemic that antibiotics have been liberally dispensed in huge quantities and quite unnecessarily. As with so much of the story of antibiotic resistance, this need never have happened if antibiotics had been used in a more careful and controlled manner.

A common gut bacterium that used to cause mild infection in the child or debilitated adult, *Escherichia coli* has now produced highly pathogenic resistant strains due to pressure from antibiotics. *E. coli* O157 produces a haemorrhagic colitis that is transmitted via improperly cooked beef and from milk and water contaminated by infected cows. This is a new disease resulting from the misuse of antibiotics by the agricultural industry.

As if these problems were not enough, a new superbug first identified in 2008 is resistant to all known current treatments. The β-lactamase enzyme that it produces destroys antibiotics, making it immune to all but colistin and tigecycline, which are only partly effective and have unpleasant side effects. What is worse is that its resistance gene can be picked up by other bacteria, transforming them into totally resistant organisms. This has already happened with *E. coli* and is likely to happen with other bacteria, rendering the administration of antibiotics a useless strategy.

New methods will need to be tried, such as using bacteria that do us no harm to attack other bacteria, much in the same way that lactobacilli do in our intestines. In a similar manner, bacteriophages have been used for some time in typing organisms, but they could be used to destroy bacteria if a safe means of using them can be developed. The bacteriophage is a virus that preys on bacteria, injecting its DNA to make the bacterium produce large quantities of the virus and at the same time destroying it. But this clearly is a risky strategy as the bacteriophage might instead attack human cells.

Now we know about the self-destruction of cells, it may be possible to introduce genes into bacteria to cause them to commit programmed self-death.

The other approach is to protect existing antibiotics by coating them with aptamers that prevent bacteria from disabling them. Normally, bacteria disable an antibiotic by developing enzymes that metabolize it, but an aptamer coating would prevent this from happening. It may also be possible to block the attack signal that bacteria use when they reach sufficient numbers to mount their invasion of the host.

It also seems that bees might come to our aid, as researchers at Lund University in Sweden have found that honey contains a group of 13 lactic acid bacteria that may be useful in fighting infectious diseases. MRSA seems to be no problem to them. It is likely that other naturally occurring substances used by animals to protect themselves could be of value to us, if only we can find them.

All of these methods are very much at the experimental stage and will require considerable resources to develop them. In the meantime, care in the way we use antibiotics, antiseptics and cleanliness will go a long way in combating these problems.

Epilogue

We have had a period of prolonged success in overcoming infectious diseases, such that many doctors considered them to be a problem of the past. However, this is readily seen not to be the case and we need new methods to tackle diseases. Like the parasitic worms that have successfully succeeded in living in us without due effect, we need to understand how we can more closely adapt to the way of diseases. We have discovered the benefits of public health and of simple methods of prevention, not the magic bullet that has now been spent; we need to return to these simple methods in finding out how we can more easily live with disease.

Vaccines will be the main method as immunity was developed by natural selection to protect against disease-producing organisms. But even the simple methods of hygiene and prevention are effective if applied with care.

Further into the future is the realm of speculation, but one thing that we can be certain about is that new diseases will occur, possibly from animal sources as they have done in the past, or just arise from new mutations. The era of communicable diseases is not finished. We might know how to control those diseases that have troubled us in the past, but new problems will appear and we must realize that disease has always and will continue to shape our future.

Conclusions

20

It has been a long passage from single-celled organisms, the incorporation of virus-like material and the fortuitous capture and disarming of a pathogenic bacteria to produce eukaryotic cells, to the multicelled beings that we now are. We could have been all of the same sex but the drive to outwit disease and produce variety so that individuals were better able to survive has made us male and female. Think of what we would have missed, none of those dreams of a fantasy world as teenagers, falling in love and all the romanticism that went with it, sex and the great pleasures it brings, the joy of procreation and parenthood, and a continual companionship throughout life with those of the opposite sex. None of this would have happened if it had not been for the pressure of disease on evolution. Were diseases such a bad thing?

Strangely, as well as capturing bacteria to fuel all of our cells we have also allowed retroviruses to be part of our genome to assist in our rapid development. With their greater capacity to produce mutations this has speeded up our progress. We are, therefore, not only part bacteria but also part virus as well. We have used disease-producing organisms, or they have used us, to help and develop our species into what it is.

When not welcoming potentially damaging organisms and particles, disease drove animals to defend themselves with an intricate process that we can collectively call immunity. By its complexity, we can tell that it has gone through many modifications and developments and is still continuing to do so as we meet new diseases. In itself, it has saved our species from the great plagues that threatened to wipe us out, but we have also found how to enhance it by the use of vaccination. How much simpler it is to have an injection or swallow a few drops of liquid to prevent what might happen, and to rest on the assurance that we stand a good chance not to contract an affliction, rather than go through the painful process of illness and treatment. Immunity arose because of the pressure of disease.

The history of the world is as much the history of how disease altered the course of civilizations, as the great battles we are more familiar with.

Dynasties arose because of their weakened neighbours and declined because of the devastation caused by epidemic diseases. Disease has been a negative or a positive force depending on which side you were on. Huge numbers died but were replaced by fitter, more successful people to continue the human race. Great leaders and ordinary people have been struck down in their prime, only to overcome their affliction and be enhanced by it. Some of the most profound ideas that have shaped the progress of the world have come about due to the intervention of disease. It is easy to forget the influence that disease has had on the past and the present, and will continue to do in the future.

Microorganisms are everywhere, together they make up a far greater mass than the entire human race. Many of them we need just as much as they need us. Lactobacilli protect us from the moment we are born and continue to populate our intestines throughout life. Yeast makes our bread and slime moulds clean our water, yet we attack them all with our antiseptics as though they were the enemy. Some dirt is good for us and might help prevent allergies; we are not discriminating between the good and the bad.

Those organisms that do produce disease want to exploit their own particular niche and survive, in the same way as our antecedents did. Many animals are reservoirs of disease that occasionally spill over and cause us problems, but in the animal host they cause minor or no ill effect. A balance has been achieved in which both host and competing organisms survive in a collective amnesty. There are fewer diseases in which humans are reservoirs, probably because of our shorter evolutionary history, but inevitably this will be the way we will be able to live with some of them. We have already struck a balance with many of the parasitic worms that live in our intestines, except when other conditions allow them to multiply at our expense, such as in the malnourished child. However, when this is not the case, they cause us no harm and, as is becoming increasingly realized, probably actually confer benefits. If they prevent some of the more unpleasant allergies then their continued presence might be preferable, especially as most of the time we do not even know we have them.

We have had a renaissance from infectious diseases with the discovery of antibiotics, but gradually bacteria have fought back until we are at the stage now where we have nothing that can overcome the superbugs. Fortunately, these bacteria are superior only in that they can withstand the antibiotics that we use against them, and in competition with the original strains of bacteria from which they developed, they are often not successful. It would be a painful and difficult process if we were to stop using antibiotics so that these superbugs might be killed off by other strains, but it might be the only way if we are not to see their proliferation to enormous proportions.

Seeking the magic bullet has always been the Holy Grail and for many years the antibiotics seemed to be just that, but often simpler methods, although slower in action, have been just as effective. The first attempts to produce a malaria vaccine were made in 1919, almost 100 years ago, and they still continue. Every so often, we are heartened by the news that finally a malaria vaccine has been made, but then all goes quiet and we discover that it was not effective. Perhaps a malaria vaccine will eventually be developed, or we will learn how to produce mosquitoes that can no longer become infected with *Plasmodium*, but in the meantime we can use insecticide-treated mosquito nets (ITNs). One of the worst reputations for malaria was Solomon Islands, it often being said that more Japanese died from malaria than American bullets in the great battles of Guadalcanal and Munda. But by getting people to use ITNs, malaria has been reduced to such low levels in some of the islands that it has become almost non-existent. The same strategy can be used in many other parts of the world, but poverty and lack of education prevent people from being able to lift themselves above subsistence level and use such methods.

Doing simple things and caring for our own health is preferable to relying on a central organization to always protect us. Just washing our hands, especially before we eat, can prevent a surprisingly large number of infections. The mother taking care of her children is the basis on which a health system functions. Added to this is vaccination as the child increases in age. All the time education is the means by which we learn how best to run our lives. Diseases are always with us, most of which we can prevent, but at times we will need professional help to overcome them.

Disease organisms are part of us, they have shaped and developed us ever since the first bacteria appeared on the planet. They are not the enemy, something to be conquered and got rid of. This will never happen, because as soon as we have overcome one particular organism another will evolve or transfer from another species to challenge us again. Diseases are part of our life and our creation, they are as integral a part of our being as eating or drinking. We must learn to work with them and to adjust our lives so that we can gain from their benefits as well as mourn the hardships that they bring upon us.

Resource Material and Suggested Further Reading

Mainly books and web resources are listed, with only the more important or recent scientific papers, including those that are mentioned in the text.

General Reading

Axelrod, R. (1984) *The Evolution of Co-operation*. Penguin, London.

Cavalli-Sfortza, L.L. and Feldman, M.W. (1981) *Cultural Transmission and Evolution: A Quantitative Approach*. Princeton University Press, Princeton, New Jersey.

Connolly, M.A. (ed.) (2006) *Communicable Disease Control in Emergencies: A Field Manual*. World Health Organization, Geneva, Switzerland.

Cook, G.C. and Zumla, A.I. (eds) (2008) *Manson's Tropical Diseases*, 22nd edn. Saunders Elsevier Health Sciences, Philadelphia. Online access at Expert Consult.

Crawford, D.H. (2007) *Deadly Companions: How Microbes Shaped Our History.* Oxford University Press, Oxford, UK.

Dawkins, R. (1976) *The Selfish Gene*. Oxford University Press, Oxford, UK.

Dawkins, R. (1982) *The Extended Phenotype*. Oxford University Press, Oxford, UK.

Dawkins, R. (1986) *The Blind Watchmaker*. Longman, Harlow, UK.

Ewald, P.W. (1994) *Evolution of Infectious Disease*. Oxford University Press, New York.

Fisher, R.A. (1930) *The Genetical Theory of Natural Selection*. Clarendon Press, Oxford, UK.

Gee, H. (2004) *Jacob's Ladder: The History of the Human Genome*. W.W. Norton, New York and London.

Haldane, J.B.S. (1932) *The Causes of Evolution*. Longmans, Green and Co., London.

Heymann, D.L. (2012) *Control of Communicable Diseases Manual*, 20th edn. American Public Health Association (APHA Press), Washington, DC.

Jones, S. (1993) *The Language of the Genes*. Harper Collins, London.

Lucas, A.O. and Gilles, H.M. (2002) *Short Textbook of Public Health Medicine for the Tropics*. Hodder Arnold, London.

Noah, N.D. (2006) *Controlling Communicable Disease*. Open University Press, Milton Keynes, UK.

Peters, W. and Pasvol, G. (2007) *Atlas of Tropical Medicine and Parasitology*, 6th edn. Elsevier Mosby, Philadelphia, Pennsylvania.

Ridley, M. (1999) *Genome. The Autobiography of a Species in 23 Chapters*. Harper Perennial, London.

Ridley, M. (2003) *Nature via Nurture: Genes, Experiences and What Makes Us Human*. HarperCollins, New York/Fourth Estate, London.

Trivers, R. (1985) *Social Evolution*. Benjamin Cummings, Menlo Park, California.

Warrell, D., Cox, T.M. and Firth, J.D. (eds) (2010) *Oxford Textbook of Medicine*, 5th edn. Oxford University Press, Oxford, UK.

Webber, R. (2012) *Communicable Diseases: A Global Perspective*, 4th edn. CAB International, Wallingford, UK.

Wilson, E.O. (1975) *Sociobiology: The New Synthesis*. The Belknap Press of Harvard University Press, Cambridge, Massachusetts.

Wilson, E.O (1992) *The Diversity of Life*. The Belknap Press of Harvard University Press, Cambridge, Massachusetts.

Wilson, E.O. (1998) *Consilience: The Unity of Knowledge*. Alfred A. Knopf, New York.

Wills, C.W. (1991) *The Wisdom of the Genes: New Pathways of Evolution*. Oxford University Press, Oxford, UK/Basic Books, New York.

Introduction

Darwin, C. (1839) *Voyage of the Beagle*. Henry Colburn Books, London [Published by Penguin Books, London in 1989].

Darwin, C. (1859) *The Origin of Species by Means of Natural Selection, or the Preservation of Favoured Races in the Struggle for Life*. John Murray, Edinburgh, UK.

Darwin, C. (1871) *The Descent of Man, and Selection in Relation to Sex*. John Murray, Edinburgh, UK.

Chapter 1

Daly, M. and Wilson, M. (1983) *Sex, Evolution, and Behavior*, 2nd edn. Willard Grant Press, Boston, Massachusetts.

Darwin, C. (1871) *The Descent of Man, and Selection in Relation to Sex*. John Murray, Edinburgh, UK.

Gould, S.J. (1989) *Wonderful Life: The Burgess Shale and the Nature of History*. W.W. Norton, New York and London.

Grosset, J.H. (1989) *WHO Expert Committee on Leprosy, Seventh Report*. WHO Technical Report Series No. 874, World Health Organization, Geneva, Switzerland.

Hamilton, W.D. (1996) *Narrow Roads of Gene Land. Volume 1: Evolution of Social Behaviour*. W.H. Freeman, Basingstoke, UK and New York.

Hamilton, W.D., Axelrod, R. and Tanese, R. (1990) Sexual reproduction as an adaptation to resist parasites (a review) *Proceedings of the National Academy of Sciences of the United States of America* 87, 3566–3573.

Margulis, L. (1981) *Symbiosis in Cell Evolution*. W.H. Freeman, San Francisco, California.

Margulis, L. (1998) *The Symbiotic Planet: A New Look at Evolution*. Weidenfeld & Nicholson, London.

Ridley, M. (1993) *The Red Queen: Sex and the Evolution of Human Nature*. Penguin Books, London.

Villarreal, L. (2005) *Viruses and the Evolution of Life*. ASM Press, Washington, DC.

Wagner, A. (2014) *Arrival of the Fittest: Solving Evolution's Greatest Puzzle*. Oneworld, London.

Wang, Z. and Wu, M. (2014) Phylogenomic reconstruction indicates mitochondrial ancestor was an energy parasite. *PLoS ONE* 9(10): e110685.

Web resources

www.priory.com/history_of_medicine/leprosy.htm (A history of leprosy by Savona-Ventura, C. and Buttigieg, G.G. (2009) Kings, Knights and Lepers; accessed 29 June 2015).

www.who.int/lep/en (World Health Organization Leprosy elimination home page; accessed 29 June 2015).

Chapter 2

Cann, R.L., Stoneking, M. and Wilson, A.C. (1987) Mitochondrial DNA and human evolution. *Nature* 329, 31–36.

Fasching, L., Kapopoulou, A., Sachdeva, R., Petri, R., Jönsson, M.E., Männe, C., Turelli, P., Jern, P., Cammas, F., Trono, D. and Jakobsson, J. (2015) TRIM28 represses transcription of endogenous retroviruses in neural progenitor cells. *Cell Reports* 10, 20–28. (This unlikely title describes how retroviruses affect brain development.)

Green, R.E., Krause, J., Briggs, A.W., Maricic, T, Stenzel, U., Kircher, M., Patterson, N., Li, H., Zhai, W., Fritz, M.H. (2010) A draft sequence of the Neandertal genome. *Science* 328, 710–722.

Heeny, J.L., Dalgleish, A.G. and Weiss, R.A. (2006) Origins of HIV and the evolution of resistance to AIDS. *Science* 313, 462–466.

Henshilwood, C. and Sealy, J. (1997) Bone artefacts from the Middle Stone Age at Blombos Cave, Sothern Cape, South Africa. *Current Anthropology* 38, 890–895.

Kittler, R., Kayser, M. and Stoneking, M. (2003) Molecular evolution of *Pediculus humanus* and the origin of clothing. *Current Biology* 13, 1414–1417.

Leakey, R.E. (1981) *The Making of Mankind*. Michael Joseph, London/E.P. Dutton, New York.

Maudlin, I., Holmes, P.H. and Miles, M.A. (eds) (2004) *The Trypanosomiases*. CAB International, Wallingford, UK.

Miller, G.F. (2001) *The Mating Mind: How Sexual Choice Shaped the Evolution of Human Nature*. Vintage, London.

Oppenheimer, S. (2003) *Out of Eden. The Peopling of the World*. Constable & Robinson, London.

Reader, J. (1990) *Missing Links, the Hunt for Earliest Man*, 2nd edn. Penguin, London.

Reader, J. (1998) *Africa, A Biography of the Continent*. Penguin Books, London.

Reed, D., Smith, S.L., Hammond, S.L., Rogers, A.R. and Clayton, D.H. (2004) Genetic analysis of lice supports direct contact between modern and archaic humans. *PLoS Biology* 2, 1972–1883.

Ridley, M. (1993) *The Red Queen: Sex and the Evolution of Human Nature*. Penguin Books, London.

Reich, D., Green, R.E., Kircher, M., Krause, J., Patterson, N., Durand, E.Y., Viola, B., Briggs, A.W., Stenzel, U., Johnson, P.L.F. *et al.* (2010) Genetic history of an archaic hominin group from Denisova Cave in Siberia. *Nature* 468, 1053–1060.

Roberts, A. (2009) *The Incredible Human Journey: The Story of How We Colonised the Planet*. Bloomsbury, London.

Schuster, C., Miller, W., Ratan, A., Tomsho, L.P., Giardine, B., Kasson, L.R., Harris, R.S., Petersen, D.C., Zhao, F., Qi, J. *et al.* (2010) Complete Khoisan and Bantu genomes from southern Africa. *Nature* 463, 943–947.

Stringer, C. (2011) *The Origin of Our Species*. Penguin, London.

Stringer, C. and Gamble, C. (1993) *In Search of the Neanderthals: Solving the Puzzle of Human Origins*. Thames and Hudson, London.

Trinkaus, E. and Shipman, P. (1993) *The Neandertals: Changing the Image of Mankind*. Jonathan Cape, London/Alfred A. Knopf, New York.

Wade, N. (2007) *Before the Dawn: Recovering the Lost History of Our Ancestors*. Penguin, London.

Wells, S. (2006) *Deep Ancestry: Inside the Genographic Project*. National Geographic, Washington, DC.

Wilson, E.O. (2012) *The Social Conquest of Earth*. Liveright, New York.

Chapter 3

Anderson, R.M. and May, R.M. (1982) Coevolution of hosts and parasites. *Parasitology* 85, 411–426.

Anderson, R.M and May, R.M. (1991) *Infectious Diseases of Humans: Dynamics and Control*. Oxford University Press, Oxford, UK.

Baillie, J.K., Barnett, M.W., Upton, K.R., Gerhardt, D.J., Richmond, T.A., De Sapio, F., Brennan, P.M., Rizzu, P., Smith, S., Fell, M. *et al.* (2011) Somatic retrotransposition alters the genetic landscape of the human brain. *Nature* 479, 534–537.

Chiodini, P.L., Moody, D.H. and Manser, D.W. (2001) *Atlas of Medical Helminthology and Protozoology*, 4th edn. Churchill Livingstone, Edinburgh, UK.

Clutterbuck, D. (2004) *Sexually Transmitted Infections and HIV*. Mosby-Wolfe, London.

Duffy, P.E. and Fried, M. (eds) (2001) *Malaria in Pregnancy: Deadly Parasite, Susceptible Host*. Taylor & Francis, London/Informa Healthcare, New York.

Fasching, L., Kapopoulou, A., Sachdeva, R., Petri, R., Jönsson, M.E., Männe, C., Turelli, P., Jern, P., Cammas, F., Trono, D. and Jakobsson, J. (2015) TRIM28 represses transcription of endogenous retroviruses in neural progenitor cells. *Cell Reports* 10, 20–28. (This unlikely title describes how retroviruses affect brain development.)

Gluckman, P., Beedle, A. and Hanson, M. (2009) *Principles of Evolutionary Medicine*. Oxford University Press, Oxford, UK.

Heeney, J.L., Dalgleish, A.G. and Weiss, R.A. (2006) Origins of HIV and the evolution of resistance to AIDS. *Science* 313, 462–466.

Malaria Consortium (2007) *Malaria: A Handbook for Health Professionals*. Macmillan Education, Oxford, UK.

Moalem, S. (2007) *Survival of the Sickest: The Surprising Connections Between Disease and Longevity*. HarperCollins, New York.

Muller, M. (2001) *Worms and Human Diseases*, 2nd edn. CAB International, Wallingford, UK.

Nesse, R.M. and Williams, G.C. (1994) *Evolution and Healing: The New Science of Darwinian Medicine*. Phoenix, London. (US version: *Why We Get Sick: The New Science of Darwinian Medicine*. Times Books, New York.)

Oppenheimer, S.J., Hill, A.V.S., Gibson, F.D., MacFarlane, S.B., Moody, J.B. and Pringle, J. (1987) The interaction of alpha thalassaemia with malaria. *Transactions of the Royal Society of Tropical Medicine and Hygiene* 81, 322–326.

Payne, R., Muenchhoff, M., Mann, J., Roberts, H.E., Matthews, P., Adland, E., Hempenstall, A., Huang, K.-H., Brockman, M., Brumme, Z. *et al.* (2014) Impact of HLA-driven HIV adaptation on virulence in populations of high HIV seroprevalence. *Proceedings of the National Academy of Sciences of the United States of America* 111, E5393–E5400.

Reithinger, R., Kamya, M.R., Whitty, C.J.M.. Dorsey, G. and Vermund, S.H. (2009) Interaction of malaria and HIV. *British Medical Journal* 338: b2141 (1400–1401).

Villarreal, L. (2005) *Viruses and the Evolution of Life*. ASM Press, Washington, DC.

Warrell, D. and Gilles, H.M. (eds) (2002) *Essential Malariology*, 4th edn. Arnold (Hodder Headline), London.

Webber, R. (2012) *Communicable Diseases: A Global Perspective*, 4th edn. CAB International, Wallingford, UK.

World Health Organization (2007) *Long-lasting Insecticidal Nets for Malaria Prevention: A Manual for Malaria Programme Managers*, Trial edn. Geneva, Switzerland.

Web resources

www.who.int/hiv/pub/guidelines/clinicalstaging.pdf (Interim WHO Clinical Staging of HIV/AIDS and HIV/AIDS Case Definitions for Surveillance, African Region. World Health Organization; accessed 1 July 2015).

www.who.int/tb/en (World Health Organization Tuberculosis (TB) home page; accessed 1 July 2015).

Chapter 4

Buxton, P.A. and Hopkins, G.H.E. (1927) *Researches in Polynesia and Melanesia.* Memoirs of the London School of Hygiene and Tropical Medicine No. 1, London.

Dennis, G.T., Gage, K.L., Gratz, N., Poland, J.D. and Tikhomirov, E. (1999) *Plague Manual: Epidemiology, Distribution, Surveillance and Control.* Document No. WHO/CDS/CSR/EDC/99.2, World Health Organization, Geneva, Switzerland.

Goddard, J. (2008) *Infectious Diseases and Arthropods*, 2nd edn. Humana (Springer), Totowa, New Jersey.

Halstead, S. (ed.) (2008) *Dengue.* Tropical Medicine: Science and Practice, Volume 5, Imperial College Press, London.

Pichon, G. (2002) Limitation and facilitation in the vectors and other aspects of the dynamics of filarial transmission: the need for vector control against *Anopheles*-transmitted filariasis. *Annals of Tropical Medicine and Parasitology* 96, S143–S152.

Pichon, G., Perrault, G. and Laigret, J. (1974) Rendement parasitaire chez les vecteurs de filarioses. *Bulletin of the World Health Organization* 51, 517–524. (Also Pichon, G., Perrault, G. and Laigret, J. (1975) Document non publié WHO/FIL/75.132, World Health Organization, Geneva, Switzerland.)

Service, M.W. (ed.) (2001) *The Encyclopaedia of Arthropod-transmitted Infections of Man and Domestic Animals.* CAB International, Wallingford, UK.

Wallace, A.R. (1869) *The Malay Archipelago: The Land of the Orang-utan, and the Bird of Paradise. A Narrative of Travel, with Studies of Man and Nature.* Macmillan, London.

Webber, R.H. (1991) Can anopheline-transmitted filariasis be eradicated? *Journal of Tropical Medicine and Hygiene* 94, 241–244.

Webber, R. (2012) *Communicable Diseases: A Global Perspective*, 4th edn. CAB International, Wallingford, UK.

Webber, R.H. and Southgate, B.A. (1981) The maximum density of anopheline mosquitoes that can be permitted in the absence of continuing transmission of filariasis. *Transactions of the Royal Society of Tropical Medicine and Hygiene* 75, 499–506.

World Health Organization (1992) *Lymphatic Filariasis: The Disease and its Control. Fifth Report of the WHO Expert Committee on Filariasis.* WHO Technical Report Series No. 821, Geneva, Switzerland.

World Health Organization (2007) *Long-lasting Insecticidal Nets for Malaria Prevention: A Manual for Malaria Programme Managers*, Trial edn. WHO, Geneva, Switzerland.

Youngson, P. (2001) *Jura, Island of Deer.* Birlinn, Edinburgh, UK.

Zhang, S.Q., Zhang, Q.G., Cheng, F., Wang, L.L. and Pen, G.P. (1991) Threshold of transmission of *Brugia malayi* by *Anopheles sinensis*. *Journal of Tropical Medicine and Hygiene* 94, 245–250.

Chapter 5

Crawford, D.H. (2007) *Deadly Companions, How Microbes Shaped Our History.* Oxford University Press, Oxford, UK.

Dennis, G.T., Gage, K.L., Gratz, N., Poland, J.D. and Tikhomirov, E. (1999) *Plague Manual: Epidemiology, Distribution, Surveillance and Control*. Document No. WHO/CDS/CSR/EDC/99.2. World Health Organization, Geneva, Switzerland.

Hopkins, D.R. (1983) *Princes and Peasants: Smallpox in History*. University of Chicago Press, Chicago, Illinois.

Oldstone, M.B.A. (2010) *Viruses, Plagues, and History: Past, Present, and Future*, revised and updated edn. Oxford University Press, New York.

Ranger, T. and Slack, P. (eds) (1992) *Epidemics and Ideas: Essays on the Historical Perception of Pestilence*. Cambridge University Press, Cambridge, UK.

Webber, R. (2012) *Communicable Diseases: A Global Perspective*, 4th edn. CAB International, Wallingford, UK.

Web resources

www.who.int/wer/2015/en/ (*Weekly Epidemiological Record* (*WER*) of the World Health Organization. Up-to-date information on current epidemics; accessed 1 July 2015).

Chapter 6

Coates, A. (1970) *Western Pacific Islands*. Her Majesty's Stationery Office, London.

Webber, R. (2012) *Communicable Diseases: A Global Perspective*, 4th edn. CAB International, Wallingford, UK.

Chapter 7

Mahmoud, A. (ed.) (2001) *Schistosomiasis*. Tropical Medicine: Science and Practice, Volume 3. Imperial College Press, London.

Web resources

www3.imperial.ac.uk/schisto (Schistosomiasis Control Initiative of Imperial College London; accessed 1 July 2015).

Chapter 8

Bates, H.W. (1863) *The Naturalist on the River Amazons: A Record of Adventures, Habits of Animals, Sketches of Brazilian and Indian life and Aspects of Nature Under the Equator During Eleven Years of Travel*. John Murray, London.

Darwin, C. (1839) *Voyage of the Beagle*. Henry Colburn Books, London [Republished by Penguin Books, London in 1989].

Darwin, F. (ed.) (1902) Charles Darwin. *His Life Told in an Autobiographical Chapter, and in a Selected Series of his Published Letters.* John Murray, London.

Dillehay, T.D., Ramírez, C., Pino, M., Collins, M.B., Rossen, J. and Pino-Navarro, J.D. (2008) Monte Verde: seaweed, food, medicine and the peopling of South America. *Science* 320, 784–786.

Humboldt, A. von (1907) *Personal Narrative of Travels to the Equinocital Regions of America During the Years 1799–1804, Volume II* (translated from the French of Alexander von Humboldt and edited by T. Ross). George Bell & Sons, London.

Wallace, A.R. (1889) *A Narrative of Travels on the Amazon and Rio Negro, with an Account of the Native Tribes, and Observations on the Climate, Geology, and Natural History of the Amazon Valley.* Ward Lock, London.

Chapter 9

Ewald, P.W. (1994) *Evolution of Infectious Disease.* Oxford University Press, New York.

Snow, J. (1849) *On the Mode of Communication of Cholera.* (Leaflet; 2nd much enlarged edition published in 1855 by John Churchill, London and available at: http://www.ph.ucla.edu/epi/snow/snowbook.html; accessed 1 July 2015.)

Webber, R. (2012) *Communicable Diseases: A Global Perspective*, 4th edn. CAB International, Wallingford, UK.

Web resources

www.who.int/cholera/en (World Health Organization Cholera home page, including information on the Global Task Force on Cholera Control; accessed 1 July 2015).

Chapter 10

Van-Tam, J. and Sellwood, C. (2010) *Introduction to Pandemic Influenza.* CAB International, Wallingford, UK.

Villarreal, L. (2005) *Viruses and the Evolution of Life.* ASM Press, Washington, DC.

Web resources

www.who.int/csr/disease/influenza/en (WHO Influenza home page; accessed 1 July 2015).

Chapter 11

Eckert, J., Gemmell, M.A., Meslin, F.-X. and Pawłowski, Z.S. (eds) (2001) *WHO/ OIE Manual on Echinococcosis in Humans and Animals: A Public Health*

Problem of Global Concern. World Health Organization, Geneva, Switzerland/ World Organisation for Animal Health, Paris.

Flegr, J., Havlícek, J., Kodym, P., Malý, M. and Smahel, Z. (2002) Increased risk of traffic accidents in subjects with latent toxoplasmosis: a retrospective case-control study. *BMC Infectious Diseases* 2, 11.

Macpherson, C.N., Meslin, F.-X. and Wandeler, A.L. (eds) (2000) *Dogs, Zoonoses and Public Health*, 2nd edn. CAB International, Wallingford, UK.

Webber, R. (2012) *Communicable Diseases: A Global Perspective*, 4th edn. CAB International, Wallingford, UK.

World Health Organization (2005) *WHO Expert Consultation on Rabies, First Report, Geneva, 5–8 October 2004*. WHO Technical Report Series No. 931, Geneva, Switzerland.

World Health Organization, Food and Agriculture Organization of the United Nations and World Organisation for Animal Health (2008) *Anthrax in Humans and Animals*, 4th edn. WHO, Geneva, Switzerland/FAO, Rome/OIE, Paris.

Chapter 12

Childs, J.E., Mackenzie, J.S. and Richt, J.A. (eds) (2007) *Wildlife and Emerging Zoonotic Diseases: The Biology, Circumstances and Consequences of Cross-Species Transmission*. Current Topics in Microbiology and Immunology, Volume 315. Springer, Berlin.

Webber, R. (2012) *Communicable Diseases: A Global Perspective*, 4th edn. CAB International, Wallingford, UK.

Chapter 13

Antal, G.M., Lukehart, S.A. and Meheus, A.Z. (2002) Review: the endemic tre-ponematoses. *Microbes and Infection* 4, 83–94.

Rogstad, K. (ed.) (2011) *ABC of Sexually Transmitted Infections*, 6th edn. BMJ Books, Wiley-Blackwell, Oxford and Chichester, UK.

Steel, T. (1975) *The Life and Death of St. Kilda*. Fontana (HarperCollins), Glasgow/ London.

Chapter 14

Blaser, M. (2014) *Missing Microbes: How Killing Bacteria Creates Modern Plagues*. One World, London.

van Nood, E., Vrieze, A., Nieuwdorp, M., Fuentes, S., Zoetendal, E.G., de Vos, W.M., Visser, C.E., Kuijper, E.J., Bartelsman, J.F.W.M., Tijssen, J.G.P. *et al.* (2013) Duodenal infusion of donor feces for recurrent *Clostridium difficile*. *New England Journal of Medicine* 368, 407–415.

Webber, R. (2012) *Communicable Diseases: A Global Perspective*, 4th edn. CAB International, Wallingford, UK.

Chapter 15

Cordain, L., Eaton, S.B., Miller, J.B., Mann, N. and Hill, K. (2002) The paradoxical nature of hunter–gatherer diets: meat based, yet non-atherogenic. *European Journal of Clinical Nutrition* 56(Suppl. 1), S42–S52.

Crous-Bou, M., Fung, T.T, Prescott, J., Julin, B., Du, M., Sun. Q., Rexrode, K.M., Hu, F.B. and De Vivo, I. (2014) Mediterranean diet and telomere length in Nurses' Health Study: population based cohort study. *British Medical Journal* 349: g6674.

Gluckman, P., Beedle, A. and Hanson, M. (2009) *Principles of Evolutionary Medicine*. Oxford University Press, Oxford, UK.

Trowell, H. and Burkitt, D. (eds) (1981) *Western Diseases. Their Emergence and Prevention*. Edward Arnold, London/Harvard University Press, Cambridge, Massachusetts.

Web resources

www.cdc.gov/obesity/data/adult.html (Cost of adult obesity in the USA from the Centers for Disease Control and Prevention; accessed 1 July 2015).

www.who.int/mediacentre/factsheets/fs311/en (Estimates of obesity from the World Health Organization; accessed 1 July 2015).

Chapter 16

Moalem, S. (2007) *Survival of the Sickest: The Surprising Connections Between Disease and Longevity*. Harper Collins, New York.

Parkin, D.M., Stjernsward, J. and Muir, C.S. (1984) Estimates of the worldwide frequency of twelve major cancers. *Bulletin of the World Health Organization* 62, 163–182.

Web resources

www.cancerresearchuk.org/cancer-info/cancerstats/world/incidence (Worldwide cancer incidence statistics from Cancer Research UK; accessed 1 July 2015).

www.worldlifeexpectancy.com (Life expectancy and cancer rates from World Life Expectancy, LeDuc Media; accessed 1 July 2015).

Chapter 17

Githeko, A.K, Lindsay, S.W., Confalonieri, U.E. and Patz, J.A. (2000)Climate change and vector-borne diseases: a regional analysis.*Bulletin of the World Health Organization*78,1136–1147.Available at: www.who.int/bulletin/archives/78(9)1136.pdf (accessed 1 July 2015).

Chapter 18

Childs, J.E., Mackenzie, J.S. and Richt, J.A. (eds) (2007) *Wildlife and Emerging Zoonotic Diseases: The Biology, Circumstances and Consequences of Cross-Species Transmission*. Current Topics in Microbiology and Immunology, Volume 315. Springer, Berlin.
Webber, R. (2012) *Communicable Diseases: A Global Perspective*, 4th edn. CAB International, Wallingford, UK.

Web resources

www.cdc.gov/ncidod/eid/index.htm (*Journal of Emerging Infectious Diseases* from the US Centers for Disease Control and Prevention; accessed I July 2015).
www.hpa.org.uk/Topics/InfectiousDiseases/InfectionsAZ/EmergingInfections/EmergingInfectionsMonthlySummaries/ (Emerging infections: monthly summaries. Covers new or emerging infectious disease events that could affect UK public health; published monthly by Public Health England (PHE), with the UK Department for Environment Food and Rural Affairs (Defra) and the UK Animal and Plant Health Agency (APHA); accessed I July 2015).
www.luminarium.org/encyclopedia/sweatingsickness.htm (History of the English sweating sickness from the Luminarium Encyclopedia; accessed 1 July 2015).

Chapter 19

Ridley, M. (1997) *Predictions: The Future of Disease*. Phoenix, London.
Webber, R. (2012) *Communicable Diseases: A Global Perspective*, 4th edn. CAB International, Wallingford, UK.

Web resources

www.cdc.gov/obesity/data/adult.htm (Cost of obesity in the USA from the US Centers for Disease Control and Prevention; accessed 1 July 2015).
www.who.int/mediacentre/factsheets/fs311/en (Estimates of obesity from the World Health Organization; accessed 1 July 2015).

Index

Note: Page numbers in *italics* represent tables and those in **bold** represent figures.

About the Author

Roger Webber was brought up in East Africa and read medicine at the Royal Free Hospital, London. He went out to Solomon Islands as a general medical officer, but became interested in filariasis, and set up a research project that was to keep him there for the next 10 years. The results helped to pave the way to the World Health Organization's global programme to eliminate filariasis. Having got to know the islands in such detail, he wrote down his experiences in *Solomoni: Times and Tales from Solomon Islands*.

He then went to Mbeya as the Medical Coordinator of the UK/Tanzania health project, charged with building a referral hospital and putting in health services at a time when Tanzania was ravaged by epidemics of cholera, measles and sleeping sickness. From these times *Return to Zanzibar: Travels through Africa* was written. He also began work on his textbook, *Communicable Diseases: a Global Perspective*, which was finally published after he had joined the staff of the London School of Hygiene and Tropical Medicine in 1985. Although he was mainly involved in teaching, he helped set up the new School of Public Health in Hanoi, Vietnam, as well as collaborative research projects in China, India, Nepal, Myanmar, Thailand, Indonesia, Ethiopia, Syria, Brazil and Venezuela.

After retiring to Scotland, he produced four more editions of his textbook and collaborated with an international group of contributors to publish *Maternal and Perinatal Health in Developing Countries* in 2012. He continues to travel the world as well as take a keen interest in the further education of his seven grandchildren.